Communication and Image in Nursing

Communication and Image in Nursing

Karen M. Sherman, RN, MS Ed

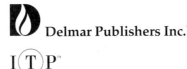

Delmar Publishers Inc.™

I(T)P™

NOTICE TO THE READER

Cover Design: J^2 Designs

Delmar Publishing Team
Publisher: David C. Gordon
Senior Acquisitions Editor: Bill Burgower
Assistant Editor: Debra M. Flis
Project Editor: Danya M. Plotsky
Production Coordinator: Barbara A. Bullock
Art and Design Coordinators: Megan K. DeSantis
                                 Timothy J. Conners

For information, address

Delmar Publishers Inc.
3 Columbia Circle, Box 15015,
Albany, NY 12212-5015

Printed in the United States of America
Published simultaneously in Canada
by Nelson Canada,
a division of The Thomson Corporation

1 2 3 4 5 6 7 8 9 10 XXX 00 99 98 97 96 95 94

Library of Congress Cataloging-in-Publication Data

Sherman, Karen M.
Communication and image in nursing / Karen M. Sherman.
    p. cm — (RealNursing series)
Includes bibliographical references and index.
ISBN 0-8273-5689-7
1. Nurse and patient. 2. Communication in nursing. 3. Nursing-Psychological aspects.
I. Title. II. Series.
[DNLM: 1. Communication—nurses' instruction. 2. Nurse-Patient Relations. WY 87 S5525c 1994]
RT86.3.S55   1994
810.73'014—dc20
DNLM/DLC   93-33352
for Library of Congress   CIP

REALNURSING SERIES
Alice M. Stein, MA, RN, Series Editor
Medical College of Pennsylvania

HEALING YOURSELF: A NURSE'S GUIDE TO SELF-CARE AND RENEWAL

COMMUNICATION AND IMAGE IN NURSING

FEAR AND AIDS/HIV: EMPATHY AND COMMUNICATION

SEXUAL HEALTH: A NURSE'S GUIDE

20 LEGAL PITFALLS FOR NURSES TO AVOID

TO LISTEN, TO COMFORT, TO CARE: REFLECTIONS ON DEATH AND DYING

THE NURSE AS HEALER

MEDICATION ERRORS: THE NURSING EXPERIENCE

FUTURE TITLES:

CRITICAL BUSINESS SKILLS FOR NURSES

HEALING ALCOHOL AND SUBSTANCE ABUSE

ETHICAL DILEMMAS IN NURSING

WAR STORIES: DIFFICULT NURSING DECISIONS

THE FEMINIST NURSE

THE GAY AND LESBIAN NURSE

INTERVENTIONS IN EVERYDAY NURSING EMERGENCIES

HEALING RACISM IN NURSING

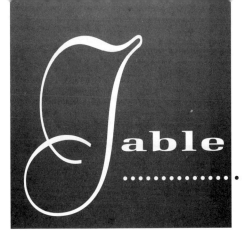

Table of Contents

PREFACE ■ xi

ACKNOWLEDGMENTS ■ xiii

CHAPTER 1 ■ 1
COMMUNICATION SKILLS

Professional Demands 2
What Is Communication? 2
Learning to Communicate 3
Summary 6

CHAPTER 2 ■ 7
EFFECTIVE COMMUNICATION

Communication Goals and Outcomes 8
Communication Models 10
One-Way Communication 11
Two-Way Communication 12
Filters 12
Verbal Communication..13
Nonverbal Communication 14
Communication Theories 16
Summary 18

CHAPTER 3 ■ 19
COMMUNICATION PROBLEMS

Whole Messages Versus Partial Messages 20
Metamessages..20
Message Busters 21
Communication and Nursing Tasks..24
Summary 26

CHAPTER 4 ■ 27
TALKING TO YOURSELF

Negative Affirmations 31
Positive Affirmations 32
Summary 35

CHAPTER 5 ■ 37
SELF-CARE

Self-Esteem: Know Thyself 39
Visualizations 40
Writing Affirmations 42
Journals 43
Spiritual Well-Being 45
Summary 48

CHAPTER 6 ■ 49
THERAPEUTIC USE OF SELF, EMPATHY, AND TRUST

Knowing the Patient 50
Therapeutic Use of Self 51
Empathy 52
Sense of Trust 54
Balanced Professional Relationships 56
Summary 58

CHAPTER 7 ■ 59
ACTIVE LISTENING

Purpose of Active Listening 61
Active Listening Skills 61
Summary 68

CHAPTER 8 ■ 69
INTERVIEWING SKILLS

Using Standard Forms 70
Information-gathering Techniques 71
Special Interviewing Challenges 74
Interviewing Errors 75
Summary 78

CHAPTER 9 ■ 79
COMMUNICATING EMOTIONS

The Sick Role 80
Putting Patients First 80
Courtesy 81
Patient Complaints 81
Emotional Support for Difficult Patients 84
Reactions to Illness 86
Summary 94

CHAPTER 10 ■ 95
COMMUNICATION CHALLENGES

Crisis Intervention 96
Suicide 98
Death and Dying 100
Communicating with Children 104
Communicating with the Elderly 106
Summary 109

CHAPTER 11 ■ 111
FAMILIES AND OTHER GROUPS

Families and Chronic Disease 112
Cultural Differences 117
Groups 119
Summary 126

CHAPTER 12 ■ 127
HUMOR AND SPIRITUALITY

Humor and Health Care 128
Spirituality 134
Spirituality and the Nurse 136
Summary 137

CHAPTER 13 ■ 139
PUBLIC SPEAKING

Professional Credibility 140
Delivery 140
Involving the Audience 141

Formal Presentations 142
Health Education 144
Using Speaking Skills 145
Summary 146

CHAPTER 14 ■ 147
PROFESSIONAL IMAGE, SHEILA M. BOYLE

What Affects the Nurse's Image?...148
A Woman's World?..149
Ways to Build Image...150
Summary 155

SUGGESTED READING ■ 157

INDEX ■ 159

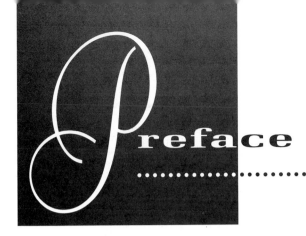

Preface

WHY NURSES NEED COMMUNICATION SKILLS

Communication and Image in Nursing is a practical book containing a number of applied concepts that work for today's nurse.

I have played a variety of nursing roles over the past 25 years and have observed many situations in which the art of communication and interpersonal relationships are most challenging. These roles included direct caregiver, clinical instructor, administrator, educator, clinical specialist, and family therapist. I will draw on these experiences throughout the book.

I have often observed health care professionals communicating with patients and saying the first thing that came to mind. Although their intentions were well-meaning, their offhand comments caused patients to respond with anger. A comment such as "Don't worry, everything will be fine," may be perceived as inappropriate by the family of a comatose patient. Some of the patients went on to repeat the story to others, and some even filed complaints with the hospital administrator.

Certain principles should guide the nurse in the area of therapeutic communication. The nurse-patient relationship is defined as an inter-action between the nurse and the patient that contributes positively to the patient's well-being. Carl Rogers defined the term "helping rela-tionship" as one in which at least one of the parties has the intent of promoting growth, improved coping, or improved functioning. These intentions are specifically related to the nurturing aspects of nursing care. The helping relationship is somewhat complex since it is colored by perceptions, affect, past experiences, anxiety, and many other factors.

Communication and Image in Nursing highlights the major points to consider in the communication process. The first three chapters are designed to provide a simple, scientific reference base. Beginning with Chapter 4, I will share critical incidents called "close-ups" from my clinical practice. These close-ups are designed to illustrate significant points related to the application of communication theory and are intended to give the reader the opportunity to look at selected interactions in actual practice. These interactions occur in the real world, so they are not intended as examples of how nurses should interact. The close-ups demonstrate the communication principles in action.

Chapter 12 addresses humor and spirituality as positive coping tools that promote communication. Chapter 13 highlights the skills commonly used in communicating with the public. Chapter 14 is the last but not the least important chapter. In this chapter, Sheila M. Boyle discusses the public image of the nurse.

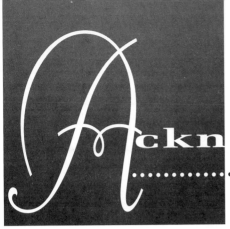

Acknowledgments

Several people have helped make this book possible. Sheila M. Boyle spent many hours reviewing and improving the manuscript. I would like to thank her for taking time out from a busy schedule to write the book's final chapter on professional image. She is truly an expert on this subject. As the nurse recruiter of Shore Memorial Hospital in Somers Point, New Jersey, Sheila guides other nurses and is an incredible model of professional behavior. She is also a supportive colleague and my humor partner.

I wish to acknowledge a few people in my life who have helped me learn about communication. Anna M. Boyle, who was my director of nursing at SUNY-Downstate Medical Center in Brooklyn, New York, taught me that process is as important as product. I thank her for teaching me about that process. I wish to pay special tribute to my mother, Anastasia T. Morris, for being the best active listener a child could ever have. I wish to express a special thanks to my father, John J. Morris, for teaching me about written language and public speaking. When I was eight, he taught me how to use a dictionary.

I owe a special thanks to my friend and colleague, Dr. Carole Zawid, whose encouragement always keeps me going. Marie Schofield and Nancy Sweger are to be credited for their high level of clerical support.

Finally, I wish to thank my husband, Arthur, and my beautiful daughters, Rachael and Anna, who are always there for me. I wish to pay special tribute to all the nurses and patients that I have known. They have helped me understand. For it is through my personal interactions with them that I know who I am and who I aspire to become.

Chapter 1

Communication Skills

Communication is a basic skill that is just as important as many other nursing skills. When nurses communicate effectively, they are valued at work, they make and keep friends, and they are respected and trusted by their family members. Your ability to communicate can contribute to your personal happiness.

This book is a guide for practicing nurses who wish to improve the way they communicate with patients, families, physicians, administrators—and also with themselves. Communicating with yourself, or "self-talk," is one skill that generates the emotional benefits needed to ensure your mental health and personal happiness. Specific communication skills enhance patient satisfaction by developing sensitivity and empathy. The skills described in this book can be applied in many different ways to improve communication at work and at home.

PROFESSIONAL DEMANDS

Because of cutbacks, job stress, an overall shortage of nurses, and health care reform, nursing today is difficult and often frustrating. Technology is more complex, families are more demanding, and nurses are expected to do more with less. Yet nursing still draws dedicated professionals who want a satisfying career in which they can help others.

The status of the nursing profession has increased as the importance of sophisticated scientific knowledge and technical skills has increased. The art of caring, which is an important part of nursing, encompasses the nurse's ability to express or engender empathy, trust, active listening, and a variety of interpersonal skills. This high-tech era of health care requires the nurse to perform technical skills proficiently. The patient, however, demands effective interpersonal skills from that same nurse. The nurse must be able to meet both of these demands so that the patient feels "cared for." This is no easy achievement. To practice nursing at this level requires discipline, balance, and commitment.

WHAT IS COMMUNICATION?

Communication is the sharing of experience. To some extent, all living organisms share experiences. However, humans are unique in their superior ability to create and use symbols. This ability enables them to share experiences indirectly and share feelings and emotions through verbal and nonverbal communication. Although communication is generally thought of as the use of words, it also includes facial expressions, eye contact, gestures, body language, and vocal cues.

Human communication is the process of creating meaning between two or more people, which can occur in a variety of situations. These situations can be placed in five broad categories to focus the analysis of human communication.

1. Two-person

2. Small group

3. Public

4. Organizational

5. Mass communication

The skills related to these categories will be developed in this book. In addition, there will be a chapter on self-talk, the use of therapeutic humor, and attention to special patient populations.

LEARNING TO COMMUNICATE

Communication is not a skill that can be taken for granted; it is a learned response that can improve with practice. There are three ways that humans learn to communicate: through conditioning, reinforcement, and modeling. Nurses are exposed to all three types in both professional and personal situations, and each type shapes the way nurses communicate in future situations.

If the nurse finds that a certain method of communication works in a given situation, it is highly likely that this method will be used again and again. But even if the nurse is satisfied with the communication, the others involved may not be. Since the goal of communication is to create meaning, it is important to determine the success of every situation.

Conditioning

Human responses are conditioned. People learn to repeat conditioned responses over and over again. Nurses are familiar with classical conditioning, demonstrated by Pavlov's experiment with the hungry dog. The dog learned to salivate in response to a signal for food rather than to the food itself. This sort of conditioned response can be observed in communication. Hearing a certain person's name can elicit a strong feeling of like or dislike. For example, the nurse who has cared for a very difficult patient may become upset and ill-tempered upon hearing this patient's name at morning report. The name is a reminder of an unpleasant experience.

Reinforcement

Learning to communicate is reinforced by rewards that increase the likelihood of repeating a specific behavior. A reward is received for giving the desired response.

B. F. Skinner demonstrated this type of learning in an experiment with hungry pigeons. The birds pecked on a box when looking for food. When they pecked at a lighted window on the box, food was received. The food was the reinforcement for giving the desired response. Soon the birds learned that to obtain food they only needed to peck at the lighted window.

Reinforcement can be observed in certain nursing situations, for example, when the nurse gives the desired response to the physician. A physician may make an unreasonable request in a harsh tone of voice, expecting the nurse to say "Yes, doctor." The nurse responds as expected and is rewarded for being a good nurse. Elimination of a response by withholding reinforcement is called extinction. For example, this same nurse may decide to extinguish this type of harsh communication by being neither sweet nor compliant. She might respond with an assertive answer such as "Excuse me, doctor, I will take orders from you when you speak in a reasonable tone of voice." The nurse is giving a direct and honest expression of her feelings and beliefs. Once the nurse acquires a new, appropriate response, it can then be generalized to other difficult situations. Without the ability to generalize, it would be impossible to develop communication skills.

All social situations depend upon our ability to discriminate and react selectively. Discrimination is the ability to learn that a response has different consequences in different situations. Humans learn to select the communication that is best suited for each situation.

Modeling

We learn many of our responses through modeling, or imitation, which begins at a very early age. In observing our parents, we learn to communicate by imitating their facial expressions and body language. As we come in contact with others, we select responses and adapt them over time. We continue to use modeling throughout our lives. Nurses use modeling when they imitate an instructor or supervisor they knew when they were students; they want to be the kind of nurse that this person exemplified. It is interesting to note that some early nursing leaders were similar in personality and style.

Mass communication makes it possible to be influenced by a particular type of style. Through television and magazines, we are given messages of how the healthy American man or woman should look and act. We are also influenced in the way we think about certain global issues. If the media has utilized effective communication techniques, we have received the message intended. Mass communication is very powerful because it affects millions of people.

Practicing Communication

Communication skills can be learned in the same way other skills are learned. Through study and practice, the nurse gains proficiency in different techniques that enhance communication. These skills can be practiced during the delivery of care. When communication skills are effective, the nurse gains the satisfaction of knowing that she responded to the patient's needs like a *caring* practitioner. Each nurse enters the field with this intention, only to find that putting communication skills together with other nursing skills takes even *more* skill. After reading this book, you are encouraged to practice the communication skills described.

Summary

In this chapter, we have discussed communication as a basic skill necessary for nurses motivated by both consumer and professional demands. Human communication is the process of creating meaning between two people that must be learned through conditioning, reinforcement, and modeling. Communication skills can be learned through study and practice. They can improve communication both at work and at home.

Chapter 2

Effective Communication

Communication is effective when the stimulus, or message, initiated by the sender corresponds closely with the stimulus perceived and responded to by the receiver. We rarely reach this perfect definition. We can, however, come close to it.

COMMUNICATION GOALS AND OUTCOMES

Effective human communication includes several goals and subsequent outcomes, such as:

- promoting understanding

- bringing pleasure

- influencing attitudes

- improving relationships

- getting action

Promoting Understanding

If the receiver has an accurate understanding of the message the sender has tried to convey, we say that the communication is effective. Failures in communication are failures to achieve accuracy in content.

Bringing Pleasure

Communication is often intended to ensure a sense of well-being or to maintain human contact. Some of our brief exchanges with others, such as "Hi" or "How are you," are used to determine the well-being of others. This type of communication exchange is reassuring to both the nurse and the patient and brings pleasure to both the sender and the receiver.

Influencing Attitudes

Understanding someone's message does not necessarily mean that you agree with it. Communication is therefore used to influence attitudes. This social influence is just as important in small groups as it is in mass communication. The nurse is viewed as a change agent who, by virtue of her professional role, can and does influence others. Nurses are using their power of persuasion more effectively today because nursing leaders are heavily promoting the image of the nurse in academic programs and professional organizations. These leaders portray the public image of the nurse as strong, intelligent, and knowledgeable. Their image is worth studying in an effort to gain a new perspective.

One of the most powerful positions in the health care reform movement can be assumed by nurses, who actively utilize mass communication to send persuasive messages to the lay public. Nurses who
write editorials to local newspapers, write journal articles, or take
advantage of television media realize this powerful influence. They can
influence health care reform to benefit patients. These nurses use public communication to influence both the nursing and lay community.

Improving Relationships

Another important goal of communication is improved relationships.
Human relationships are often affected by mistrust because a message
is not understood. This is known as a primary failure in communication. So another message must be sent to improve the relationship.
Secondary failures in communication come from misunderstandings
that are often the result of anger, confusion, or frustration in failing to
understand the message as it was intended.

A primary failure occurs when a physician chooses the word "tumor"
to describe a patient's cancer diagnosis in order to soften the message.
The patient does not receive a clear and accurate message because the
physician has failed in the sending. A secondary failure can occur
when either the sender or the receiver are emotionally upset. A patient
who is highly anxious awaits the results of a biopsy. When the physician reports to the patient that he has cancer, the message is not
understood, since the patient tells his nurse that he still does not
understand his diagnosis.

Understanding a person's motivation is an important factor to consider
in the transmission of the message. The better the communication
between people, the better the relationship is likely to be.

Getting Action

A goal of some communications is to get the receiver to take action. This
is often difficult to achieve: It is easier to get the receiver to understand
your message than to agree with it. If the receiver voluntarily performs
the action desired, it means that an attitude change has occurred.

In order for action to occur, the relationship between two people
should be comfortable and symmetrical, and the receiver must agree
that the sender's request is legitimate. The sender must be able to communicate the request so that the receiver understands it.

A receiver's difficulty in understanding the message is often com-
pounded in organizational settings, such as hospitals. For example,

nurses often become frustrated when trying to get their message across to hospital administration. A simple message like "understaffed" does not get through organizational channels fast enough for the fatigued nurse. By the time it does get through, burnout has usually occurred, causing staff apathy.

Mass communication often complicates patient care issues. News broadcasts on controversial subjects like living wills, immunizations, mammography, and environmental carcinogens certainly inform the lay public but often confuse people and increase their anxiety.

Your communications can be classified by the outcome that is achieved, such as promoting understanding, bringing pleasure, influencing attitudes, improving relationships, and getting action. It's important to remember that some communications will result in more than one outcome.

COMMUNICATION MODELS

Communication can be analyzed by using a model to highlight its essential components, namely, the source, message, channel, receiver, and feedback. This analysis helps us to understand the complex process of communication so that we can increase our awareness of what works and what does not. Each of us selects a personal style of communication based on our own listening, seeing, and feeling. One of the most common models of communication is shown in Figure 2-1.

Figure 2-1
Communication Models

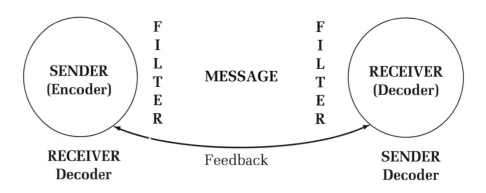

The Sender

The person who sends the message is called the sender or the source encoder. Encoding is the ability to select and use specific signs and symbols to transmit a message. The use of a particular language is the best example of encoding. A Hispanic patient's message can be accurately understood by a nurse who can understand Spanish.

The Source

The source is an idea, event, or situation. It is communicated by encoding. For example, the nurse as the encoder might ask, "Did the medication relieve your pain?" This question is actually the source or the idea to be communicated.

The Receiver

The person who receives the message is known as the decoder. Through hearing, seeing, and feeling, the decoder analyzes the message. The model in Figure 2-1 describes a communication taking place between two people. Both people are considered senders and receivers because they both send and receive messages in the course of the conversation.

The Channel

The channel is the medium through which the message is sent. Three channels that are commonly used are hearing, seeing, and feeling. When the nurse asks the patient, "Did the medication relieve your pain?" the patient hears the nurse but may also see and feel the nurse's presence.

Feedback

Feedback is the receiver's reaction to the message. For example, if a patient responds by telling the nurse that the pain medication did not work, the nurse must then react to this feedback.

ONE-WAY COMMUNICATION

Most communication is interactive and depends on both the sender and receiver. In one-way communication, the flow of information is *from* the sender *to* the receiver. One-way communication is passive and is not the best choice if the sender is interested in the receiver's response. Examples of useful one-way communication include giving shift reports and announcing that visiting hours are over. In such instances, the sender neither anticipates nor requires a response from the receiver. One-way communication is usually selected in situations in which the sender wishes to maintain control.

It may also be used inadvertently, for example, when the nurse is very busy and time does not allow for the luxury of a patient's response. Nurses may transmit the message of being too busy when they appear rushed in the presence of patients. Even if the nurse asks the patient, "Do you have any questions?" the nonverbal message transmitted is "I'm too busy to answer your questions."

TWO-WAY COMMUNICATION

Two-way communication allows and expects the receiver to give feedback and become actively involved. The receiver becomes a sender and the original sender becomes a receiver, thereby creating this two-way process. It is an active process in which the sender is able to check the receiver's understanding of the message.

The back-and-forth flow of communication is called *interaction*. The interaction between the nurse and the patient should be analyzed to measure the effectiveness of the communication. If the patient does not understand why the nurse is performing a certain procedure or treatment, it is because the nurse did not send a message that the patient could understand. When the patient receives and understands the message, the nurse can safely assume that the message was clearly communicated.

FILTERS

Filters are screens that block out parts of messages and often distort or change the message. Both the sender and the receiver filter the information that is sent and received. The sender may not be clearly communicating the message. For example, if the message is bad news, such as a deterioration in the patient's condition, the sender might find it difficult to inform the immediate family of this status change. The nurse may decide to soften the message to a family by not using accurate words to describe a patient's problem.

The family is also using a filter. They are probably anxious and are unable to receive a message that their family member is critically ill, so they only hear part of the message. The receiver's filter blocks out parts of the message. If both the sender and the receiver are using filters, only a portion of the message will get through. Filters may be conscious or unconscious, depending on the situation. The nurse or the patient may be selective during the communication. The more distorted the message is, the more filters are employed.

Filters are used in all communications. The next time you are analyzing an unsuccessful communication, try to identify the filters that were used by both the sender and the receiver.

VERBAL COMMUNICATION

Only about 7% of the total impact of a message is attributed to words. The remaining 93% of the message is nonverbal and includes facial expressions, eye contact, hand gestures, body language, and vocal cues.

The choice of words used for the verbal portion of a message is critical. The words we select come from our background and experience. If words referred only to objects, communicating would be quite easy. But words also refer to events, qualities, concepts, actions, relationships, and feelings. People assign meaning to words.

The meaning of a word is not inherent; a word gains meaning only after being associated with some reference. The primary association that a word has for most people is its denotation, or its literal meaning. Connotation, on the other hand, is the secondary association a word has for people. Sometimes, a word's connotation relates solely to one person's experience. Positive connotations stimulate positive emotions, just as negative connotations produce negative emotions. In our society, the word "housewife" often has a negative connotation. If a person has had a negative experience with a nurse, the word "nurse" may then have a negative connotation; a positive experience with a nurse will likely elicit a positive connotation.

The meaning of words can change depending upon their context and the geographic area. Words have different meanings in different areas of the country. For instance, a Harris drip may be a meaningful term for a nurse practicing in southern New Jersey but have no meaning for a nurse practicing in northern Pennsylvania.

Different cultures and subcultures have their own meanings for words. Cardiovascular nurses use terminology that cannot be understood by orthopedic nurses. Nurses who are new to a specific nursing unit must learn the language of that unit.

Communicating between two cultures can be quite complex if the two speak different languages. People who speak other languages use other symbols to represent the same words. If a person cannot translate pictures into symbols that are understood by the other culture, the communication is severely impaired, and these two parties can become frustrated.

NONVERBAL COMMUNICATION

Facial Expressions

Facial expressions are the single most important source of nonverbal communication. We constantly read expressions from other people's faces. The comment "if looks could kill" indicates the significance of facial cues.

It is considered harsh and unfair when first meeting people to judge them by their appearance. The expression "Don't judge a book by its cover" is telling us not to judge a person by how he looks. But what do we see when we look at a person's face, for example? What do we see that makes us know that the person is happy or sad? How do we know that a person is frightened or angry? By isolating facial cues, the observer can read these kinds of emotions.

Facial cues are expressions of particular emotions. To a large extent, expressive facial cues are constant across all cultures. The face has the ability to convey a wide range of emotions. An ancient Chinese proverb states: "To see a person's face is better than to hear of his reputation." This wise saying pays tribute to the face's capacity to inspire trust or raise doubt in the mind of the observer.

Eye Contact

Eye contact is a valuable source of information. It tells much about a person's personality. Because we have greater control of the muscles of the lower part of the face than we do around the eyes, the eyes can reveal the spontaneous or true response of a person. Embarrassment, guilt, fear, or anger can be discerned in others simply through eye contact.

The person who meets your eyes directly transmits a different message than the person who cannot look directly at you. When you look at someone and they shift their eyes away, you feel that he or she is avoiding you or may feel too uncomfortable with you to make eye contact.

Some cultures believe that it is disrespectful and improper to look directly into another person's eyes. However, in other cultures, a person's lack of eye contact is interpreted as a sign of dishonesty or shiftiness.

Hand Gestures

Hand gestures add another important dimension to nonverbal communication. Some people talk with their hands and these gestures can communicate their moods. Instructions to do something can be transmitted solely by using the hands, for example, through sign language. The signals used in sign language are arbitrarily chosen, and the same signals can have quite a different meaning in another culture. To an American, making the hand gesture of a circle formed by the thumb and forefinger transmits the message "Okay!" To a Brazilian, it is an obscene sign of contempt. A handshake is another gesture that transmits meaning. A limp handshake may convey a lack of interest or confidence. A damp handshake may be a sign that the person is nervous or stressed.

Body Language

Facial expressions and body language make up over 50% of the nonverbal message. Often, body language is more reliable than a verbal message. An example is the person who says, "I'm okay" but whose body language transmits "I'm not okay." The verbal message and the nonverbal message are incongruent, and the observer is convinced by the body language that something is wrong. When you are aware of this incongruence, you become a better communicator.

Body movements convey many different messages. Quick jerky movements, folding one's arms, standing rigidly, or a slumped posture all convey different meanings. If you look away as someone is talking to you, you may convey the message that you do not want to talk. Leaning away suggests that you are closed off and uninterested. If you lean toward the person, you are anxious to talk. Leaning forward can also mean that you are uncomfortable and defensive. A relaxed posture suggests that you are comfortable and open.

Vocal Cues

Vocal cues transmit a message along with the verbal message. This type of cue includes pitch, resonance, articulation, tempo, volume, and rhythm. Through vocal cues, you transmit mood and attitudes. Vocal cues convey meaning by using sounds to supplement words in the delivery of a message. The receiver may have to interpret both the sounds and the silence of the sender. For example, the nurse pauses and listens to a patient's heart with a stethoscope and says "H'mm." The patient asks, "Is something wrong?"

Sounds accompany words during the delivery of a message. Raising the pitch of the voice may be interpreted as surprise or stress. Sounds can emphasize words and clarify the meaning of the message. Sighs, throat clearing, hisses, gasps, and yawns are examples of sounds that we often use and interpret in sending messages. The inability to vocalize impairs communication. For example, the laryngectomy patient is usually frustrated and upset until he or she learns how to speak.

COMMUNICATION THEORIES

There are many theories regarding communication and interpersonal relationships for nurses. Three theorists that have practical application are Peplau, King, and Satir.

Peplau

In 1951, Hildegard Peplau wrote the first book on the interpersonal process and nursing. She identified something called the therapeutic interpersonal process, which required two or more persons in the communication. Peplau believed that a successful communication should have clarity and continuity.

Both the sender and the receiver should clearly understand the meaning of the message. The nurse is responsible for continuity by recognizing the therapeutic needs of the patient during the course of the conversation. The nurse identifies these needs by listening, feeling, and seeing.

It should be clearly understood that patients usually do not state all their needs verbally. Often, the nurse uses intuition to recognize a patient's need; the nurse is extremely aware of particular needs and just "knows" that a problem or need should be addressed. Peplau advocated the use of open-ended questions, clarification, and validation in determining needs. These skills will be addressed in later chapters.

King

Imogene King discussed communication theory as it relates to nursing. She focused her theory on the interaction between the patient and the nurse. She believed that interaction is a process of perception between a person and his or her environment. She thought of people as "open systems" that interact with the environment.

King described three separate systems that need to be acknowledged in the care of the patient: the personal system, the interpersonal system, and the social system.

The personal system is the patient's own perception, body image, growth and development, time, and space. Intrapersonal communication, such as self-talk, is important in relation to the personal system.

The interpersonal system consists of two or more individuals relating to one another. The interpersonal system takes into account roles, interactions, communication, and stress. It is through perceptions of verbal and nonverbal communication and the environment that interactions occur. Successful interactions are sought by the nurse in the interest of fostering positive interpersonal relationships with the patient.

Social systems are also important for the nurse to consider. King defines social systems as any group with a special interest that can collectively form an organization, such as the family or the hospital. Social systems in our society are family systems, religious or belief systems, educational systems, and work systems. When the nurse communicates with the patient's family, he or she is interacting with a social system.

Satir

Virginia Satir described communication style by assessing congruence. Congruence is the study of how well verbal language, body language, tone, facial expressions, and all other elements of communication fit together. A common example of a lack of congruence is the patient who states "I'm fine," while holding his abdomen and grimacing. This patient does not wish to communicate that he is in pain.

Satir also believed that feelings of self-worth impact communication. Positive self-worth can be a great asset. We rely on others' reactions to us. If you are feeling down about yourself, this feeling is often reflected in your communication with others. You begin to believe that other people think you are as worthless as you are feeling at that moment. Satir also linked self-worth with stress. She believed that we experience stress when our self-worth is compromised.

Summary

Communication is effective when the message initiated by the sender corresponds closely with the response of the receiver. The goals of communication include bringing pleasure, influencing attitudes, improving relationships, and getting action. Communication can be analyzed by a model that highlights the essential components, such as source, message, channel, receiver, and feedback. Communication may be one way or two way. Most communication is interactive and dependent upon both a sender and a receiver. All communications contain filters or screens that change or distort the message. These filters may be conscious or unconscious and are used by both the sender and the receiver. Only about 7% of the total message depends on verbal communication, with the rest of the message being sent through nonverbal communication. Facial expressions, eye contact, hand gestures, body language, and vocal cues are types of nonverbal communication.

Chapter 3

Communication Problems

Communication skills can build or repair bridges between ourselves and others. Without these bridges, we may be cut off from people who are important to us. We must be aware of our unconscious patterns of communication that negatively impact upon our interactions. This chapter will highlight common problems associated with communication.

WHOLE MESSAGES VERSUS PARTIAL MESSAGES

Whole messages include what you see, feel, think, and need. Whole messages do not leave out your feelings or cover the fact that you may be very angry. When something is left out of a message, it becomes partial or incomplete. Every situation or relationship, however, does not require a complete message. When a partial message omits something important, the message becomes obscured or distorted, and your intended meaning is lost.

METAMESSAGES

There are often two levels of meaning in a message. On one level is the information being communicated by words. On another level, the sender is communicating attitudes and feelings, or metamessages, by using some of the nonverbal elements discussed in Chapter 2. Nurses are often the receivers of metamessages from patients, family members, and physicians. A family member may state, "My mother needs a nurse who can take care of her properly." A nurse who receives such a message might determine that the family is not only demanding expert nursing care but questioning the nurse's ability. The nurse walks away feeling angry and inferior.

If the nurse tuned in to the metamessage, she may realize that the family member wanted the best for the patient and may have been feeling helpless. By displacing this feeling onto the nurse, the family member momentarily feels better.

Metamessages are the source of much interpersonal conflict. Negative metamessages communicate emotions such as blame and anger, and it can be difficult to defend yourself against the feelings they engender. However, it is possible to recognize your own metamessages and also deal with the negative metamessages of others. In subsequent chapters, we will look at specific strategies that can make a difference in improving both our own messages and those we receive from patients and families.

MESSAGE BUSTERS

There are several blocks, or "messages busters," that can prevent a message from being communicated completely. The following message busters block messages:

- Excessive talk

- Judging

- Advising

- Arguing

- Derailing

- Placating

- Inferiority/Defensiveness

- Incongruence

- False reassurance

- Distraction

- Too busy

Excessive Talk

You may have tried to send a message to someone while they were sending a message to you. Or, when that person was speaking to you, you were thinking about what you were going to say next. Discomfort with silence is another potential message buster. Because some people are uncomfortable with silence, they feel compelled to talk and talk and talk. Such talk is usually not important to the message, and it does not allow time for reflection and exploration of thoughts.

Judging

When you prejudge speakers, perhaps by deciding they are crazy or unqualified, you are not going to pay attention to the message they are attempting to convey. When nurses make judgments about patients, it can be extremely detrimental to their communication. For example, a patient may be labeled as a hypochondriac, and although she conveys the message of feeling ill, she will be ignored. A judgment should be made only after hearing and evaluating the content of a message.

Advising

Giving advice is often viewed as a part of the nurse's role. When someone identifies you as the nurse, he will seek you out for advice. You may feel pressured to have an answer for each person who approaches you. And because you are programmed to have the answers, you may feel compelled to answer before the person is finished speaking. You may be trying so hard to satisfy someone with the right advice that you miss the message that is being conveyed. You do not hear the feelings or the pain being expressed. The person feels isolated and lonely because you have not tried to connect on an emotional level.

Arguing

Arguing is a major block in communication. Neither party can be heard because they are too busy arguing with each other. Perhaps you have a strong need to always be right or to continually prove yourself. This need will have a negative impact on your ability to listen. You will be expressing your beliefs so emphatically that you dismiss the other person's point of view.

Derailing

Derailing, or changing the subject, is a block used by the person who has difficulty listening to a message. By derailing the speaker, the listener no longer has to deal with a painful or uncomfortable subject. Sometimes jokes serve as derailers in the conversation by making light of the topic. A patient may be sending a very serious message to his physician, who responds by making a joke and dismissing the serious nature of the question. Because the doctor is uncomfortable, she decides to block the conversation. The patient is left feeling that the doctor does not care about his concerns.

Placating

When you agree with everything a person tells you, you may be placating rather than really listening to what is being said. Placating responses are statements like "Yes!" and "Really!" and "Right!" If you find yourself using these responses several times during a conversation, you are not really listening, you are blocking. Look within yourself to determine why you would choose to block the conversation. Perhaps you do not want to be involved in the conversation or have difficulty with the subject matter or no interest in the speaker.

Inferiority/Defensiveness

If a sender transmits a feeling of superiority, the receiver will most likely feel inferior. This inferiority leads to defensiveness. The receiver is put on guard and feels unsafe. The receiver may also feel that he is being manipulated and will resist. Defensiveness is often a part of communication between the nurse and a physician who transmits superiority. Physicians may also exude a feeling of certainty; they are absolutely certain that they are right. As a result, the nurse may feel wrong and inferior.

When there is a willingness to work collaboratively, balance is reestablished in the nurse-physician relationship. When this occurs, the nurse will feel less defensive, and the physician will feel less superior.

In some situations, the nurse may wish to be viewed as superior. Putting people down is a way of blocking another person's point of view. "War stories" (that is, nurses sharing their work experiences) sometimes serve the purpose of demonstrating superiority. They also can be used to block another person from talking.

Incongruence

Incongruence is transmitting a message that does not match one's feelings. In other words, the message is false. Although a person may be aware of the real message, she may feel reluctant to express it. The sender may feel that the receiver is not ready to hear the message, or the sender may not be ready to discuss it. The timing may not be appropriate; even in transmitting messages, there is a time and a place for everything. If rapport has not yet been established, there is no trust in the relationship. Without trust, many sensitive messages cannot be revealed.

False Reassurance

While reassurance is often viewed by the nurse as an important and comforting communication tool, it can also be a communication block. Telling the patient, "Everything is going to be okay!" may seem consoling. The nurse walks away feeling that something therapeutic was done to allay the patient's anxiety. But often this type of statement minimizes the patient's anxiety and blocks any further communication. The patient's concerns are not addressed, and there is no further opportunity for discussion.

Distraction

The environment may be very distracting to communication. Noisy hallways, hot rooms, or unpleasant smells may all interfere with the transmission of a message. A common distraction in hospitals is the intercom system. The nurse and the patient are about to begin a meaningful conversation when the nurse is paged. The message is blocked, and communication does not take place.

Too Busy

Nurses are seen as (and in fact are) very busy people, and this can serve as a communication block. A patient may hesitate to bother the nurse even if there is a need to communicate. Such patients are sometimes labeled "good patients." But the good patients end up holding all their feelings inside. The "busy" behavior demonstrated by the nurse acts to block communication. As a nurse, you may even feel guilty when you sit down next to a patient's bed to talk. You may not want the other nurses to see this. Sitting down may be interpreted as a sign of tiredness or laziness. Nurses often feel that unless they are performing specific tasks, they are not doing their jobs.

COMMUNICATION AND NURSING TASKS

High-Visibility Tasks

These tasks are easily noticed by others and are often the ones for which the nurse receives recognition. High-visibility tasks are the psychomotor tasks that all nurses learn. Following procedures, filling out forms, and controlling the environment are some of the high-visibility tasks that nurses perform. When a nurse performs a high-visibility task, the outcome can be measured. For instance, the nurse administers an antipyretic to the patient, and within the hour the patient's temperature decreases by one degree. The patient feels better, the family is relieved, and the nurse feels that he did his job well.

Low-Visibility Tasks

Low-visibility tasks are not easily noticed by others. They usually involve cognitive or affective skills. Patient education and counseling are both considered low visibility and are sometimes referred to as "fluff." Nurse counselors and educators may feel less valued by others in the nursing profession. For instance, critical care nurses may view nurse counselors as nurses who "do nothing" all day. However, low-visibility tasks are client-centered and are valued highly by patients and families.

High-Visibility/Low-Visibility: A Perfect Blend

The challenge to the practicing nurse, regardless of the visibility of the tasks performed, is clear: Communication must be used effectively in all kinds of tasks.

High-visibility tasks are usually psychomotor or procedural. The nurse is expected to be able to perform the task with proficiency and skill, without harming the patient. The task may not require communication. The nurse knows how to do the procedure and has practiced it on many patients. The nurse is not anxious because she knows what to expect. The patient, on the other hand, does not know what to expect.

An example of a high-visibility task that requires clear communication is the administering of a barium enema preparation to a patient who did not know that he was to receive it. The patient will likely tell you that he is not going to cooperate. The nurse should stop the procedure and listen to the patient explain that the doctor never told him about the test. At this point, effective communication is essential. The low-visibility task must be performed in order for the high-visibility task to be completed.

An integrated approach that blends both high-visibility and low-visibility tasks is achievable. Once the beginning nurse becomes proficient in high-visibility tasks, she can then begin to master patient-centered communication skills. It is not an easy task to address both the physical and the psychological needs of patients, but it is possible and desirable.

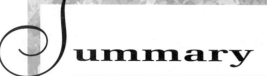

Summary

Whole messages contain what one sees, feels, thinks, and needs. When something is left out, the message is partial or incomplete. Metamessages communicate the attitudes or feelings of the sender. Messages can be blocked by excessive talk, judging, advising, arguing, derailing, placating, inferiority and defensiveness, incongruence, false reassurance, distraction, and being too busy. High-visibility tasks are easily noticed by others; low-visibility tasks are not. The challenge to practicing nurses is to communicate effectively while performing all types of tasks.

Chapter 4

Talking to Yourself

An old Chinese proverb states that "Great thoughts come from the heart." But it is just as true to say that bad thoughts come from the heart, as well. For example, when you tell yourself, "I can't do anything right," you are decreasing your self-esteem with negative self-talk. Let's take a look at an example.

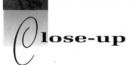

lose-up

The Student Nurse Who Would Never Amount to Anything

Susan was a senior nursing student in an urban university hospital setting. She was beautiful and caring and provided bedside nursing with a smile and a warm disposition. However, one of her nursing instructors thought that Susan could stand some toughening up. Because it was senior year and graduation was at hand, the instructor decided to put a lot of pressure on Susan to change. Susan began to crumble under the pressure, until one day the instructor told her that she would never make it as a nurse.

I was Susan's clinical instructor for her final leadership clinical rotation. I often observed her with her head down, making no eye contact. She seemed depressed and distant. One day I asked her what was bothering her. She replied, "I'm never going to make it as a nurse." Susan had begun to believe the prediction of the previous instructor.

ANALYSIS

Obviously, Susan's negative self-talk began to engulf her. Why? Each time you repeat negative phrases to yourself, you are reducing your self-esteem. The practice of negative self-talk is actually self-destructive: You lower your self-image through your own criticism and begin to see yourself as a failure.

Whether or not we realize it, each of us carries in our mind an "inner tape." This complex tape contains our lifetime of images and messages, shaped by our own thoughts and beliefs about ourselves. It records images of what we see and what others say about us. Most of all, it records our self-talk.

The practice of positive self-talk is the key to positive self-esteem. In order to feel good about ourselves and the work we do, we must send positive thoughts *to* ourselves *about* ourselves. It's important to remind ourselves about our good attributes and accomplishments.

I recently discovered two wonderful exercises to assist us in recognizing our own good work: The Standing Ovation and the Pat on the Back.

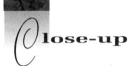

lose-up

Standing Ovation

Dana and Liz, along with two other nurses, were scheduled to work the day shift on a 32-bed medical-surgical unit. The other nurses both called in sick, leaving Dana and Liz to cover the unit themselves. The shift was a nightmare, with three pre-ops and a cardiac arrest. When their shift was over, they went to the nurses lounge and congratulated themselves: Liz gave Dana a standing ovation while Dana took a bow and smiled; then Liz did the bowing and Dana the applauding.

ANALYSIS

This close-up demonstrates a positive step that nurses can take to prevent themselves from feeling a letdown, which can lead to burnout. Dana and Liz did not wait for someone else to compliment them. While it's certainly nice to see thank-you letters from patients, they come too late to be effective. For immediate feedback, you can ask one of your colleagues to give you a standing ovation when you really need it. It is important to feel a sense of achievement before you leave for the day, to minimize that "letdown" feeling that can follow you home. A standing ovation is also a nice message of appreciation to a colleague who has put in a grueling day. This exercise encourages positive self-talk.

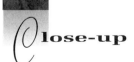

lose-up

Pat on the Back

Jan was a clinical specialist in a community hospital. She also worked with staff and was a patient advocate, which meant she had to confront physicians regarding inadequate pain control for terminally ill patients.

One afternoon, Jan had a heated discussion with a physician who resisted increasing a patient's pain medication because he felt that the patient was becoming addicted. After a very stressful confrontation, the physician finally relented and ordered the dose to be increased. Jan felt a sense of satisfaction and victory but felt she could not show this in front of the physician. So she slipped into the closest nurses lounge, stood in front of the bathroom mirror, and said, "Jan, you did a great job!"

ANALYSIS

Why did Jan compliment herself? This Pat on the Back was an *affirmation*: a positive thought or idea that consciously focuses a person to produce a desired result. Repeating affirmations is a powerful technique. In Jan's case, she had already produced the desired result. She was able to influence the physician to order the medication to be increased!

Affirmations are based on three principles:

1. Your outer reality is a direct reflection of your inner thoughts and beliefs.

2. If you change your thoughts, you change your reality.

3. Your thoughts are reflected in the written and spoken word.

Affirmations can be used to shape your inner and outer reality, or to bring a desired change into your life. Nurses often believe that they do not deserve to be loved or cared for. Perhaps they came from families in which they assumed the role of caretaker in early childhood. In dysfunctional or alcoholic families, for example, a parental child often emerges to take care of the parents and younger children.

If you find yourself saying "I do not deserve love," you may have learned this negative affirmation as a child. A positive affirmation is needed to replace this attitude. You must learn to say "I deserve love!" and you must learn to say it with conviction.

There is an affirmation for every need. You should select an affirmation that will help you to grow in a specific area, and then repeat it to yourself when you are in a relaxed state. These positive suggestions help us to reach our potential and exceed our expectations, as well as to develop a positive self-image and promote self-confidence.

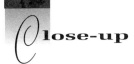

*C*lose-up

Self-Defeat

Joan was a fairly inexperienced nurse who was also accident prone. Things always seemed to happen to her. For example, on the way to work one morning, she slipped and fell in a puddle in the parking lot. Then, as she entered the hospital, she slid across the lobby and wrenched her back. As she ran to the elevator, the door closed in her face. Finally, when Joan arrived on the unit, she was met by her supervisor, who scolded her for being ten minutes late. She thought to herself, "It's not my day! No day is *ever* my day."

Joan very wearily began her workday. She was weak and tearful as she cared for her patients and could not wait until the shift ended. After work, she got into her car, only to find that the battery was dead. She had left her car lights on all day. She said, "What a klutz I am!" and began to cry. She sat in the car and thought about how right her mother was when she told her, "What a klutz you are, Joan! You never do anything right!"

ANALYSIS

Joan's problem seems so elementary. But self-defeat, especially when ingrained with messages from one's past, is a difficult attitude to change. Become aware of the conversations you have with yourself. Even if we don't realize it, we are constantly judging ourselves. If the result is negative self-talk, it creates a negative self-image and promotes self-defeat.

NEGATIVE AFFIRMATIONS

Your conscious mind is only the tip of your mental iceberg. The beliefs that create your inner and outer reality are located in the subconscious mind. This is where our thoughts about ourselves and our childhood memories, both positive and negative, are stored.

When Mohammed Ali professed, "I am the greatest!" his subconscious mind may have been saying "I think I am going to fail!" or "I'm a loser!" The subconscious mind can and often does contradict what we know to be true about ourselves. If we wish to be successful, we need to rid ourselves of old, negative beliefs and self-defeating thoughts.

Our subconscious beliefs can become conscious. The negative beliefs embedded in our subconscious are like negative affirmations. Negative beliefs sound like negative affirmations. Fortunately, our negative affirmations can be replaced by positive affirmations or positive self-talk.

POSITIVE AFFIRMATIONS

Positive affirmations are positive thoughts or ideas that we consciously focus on to produce a desired result. Positive affirmations can change our deepest thoughts and beliefs about ourselves, and can help us achieve specific goals in our lives. By changing our negative inner messages into positive messages, we change our outer reality. By repeating a positive affirmation in a calm, confident manner, a person can decrease fear and at the same time reprogram the subconscious mind. Our new beliefs become new behaviors.

How can you turn negative self-talk into positive self-talk? The next time you experience a failure or make a mistake, use the principle of positive self-talk by saying, "That's not like me. Next time, I'm going to get it right!" Learning to move on in your life in spite of your failure is like learning to walk. You'll fall or stumble a few times before you learn to do it right. When I was growing up, I learned that it was okay to make mistakes because of something my mother would tell me. She would always say, "That's why they put erasers on pencils." When I make a mistake today, I repeat this same affirmation. It's just one of the positive self-talk strategies that works for me.

Positive self-talk reinforces our desire to succeed. We set a goal and we fail. Then we try again, perhaps using a different strategy. Our self-talk reinforces our desire to succeed, and eventually we do. Our success and sense of achievement is something to celebrate. And we should try to create a mental image of how we look and feel when we succeed.

Positive people have these positive images of themselves. They replay memories of their successes, the compliments they received, and the things they did right. When we're tired, frustrated, or are having a bad day, it's important to use these instant replays to remind us of our successes. They can help us overcome our present problems and build our self-esteem.

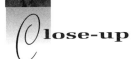

lose-up

Self Disclosure

Ann had been working on an obstetrics unit for several years. She had a miscarriage and returned to work within a few weeks. At first, Ann enjoyed being back at work, though she was a little sad when she saw the newborns through the nursery window. However, about six months later, Ann's colleagues heard her telling a patient in active labor about her miscarriage. She related the many details of this traumatic event and also told the patient that she and her husband were still trying to have a baby and would succeed!

ANALYSIS

Ann was disclosing information to a patient in what seemed to be a harmless, chatty fashion. At the time, she did not realize that this type of self-disclosure was harmful to the nurse-patient relationship. Why? Ann's self-disclosure was an attempt to make the nurse-patient relationship more real, more authentic. But by sharing this experience, she was stepping out of her nursing role and playing the role of a patient. Did this self-disclosure improve the nurse-patient relationship? The answer is obvious: Imagine yourself as the patient who was listening— you would have felt more vulnerable and possibly more afraid.

Self-disclosure should be used with care by the nurse. Certain revelations can be harmful or damaging to the nurse-patient relationship. Self-disclosure can also be an attempt to emphasize how we view our roles, rather than how others expect us to perform them. It may even be an attempt to step out of our role. When can it work? When can it improve the relationship?

Appropriate self-disclosure is not one-sided; it is a process of exchange. It should result in a buildup of trust or more positive feelings between two people. When one person discloses something, it promotes a feeling of openness and trust in the other person. How much of yourself you are willing to share with others indicates the degree of your care and support for them and affects the quality of your relationships.

The following questions can help you assess the degree of disclosure you exercise in your own life.

YES NO

___ ___ 1. I have someone in my life with whom I can talk about anything.

___ ___ 2. I keep in close touch with my extended family.

___ ___ 3. I ask for emotional support whenever I need it.

___ ___ 4. I compliment others often.

___ ___ 5. I enjoy meeting new people and do so with ease.

___ ___ 6. I can share my feelings with others at the very moment they occur.

We manage our "public" and "private" selves very differently. It is not possible to share ourselves equally with each person. However, refusing to share ourselves with anyone is likely to cause harm. What aspects of your public self are you willing to share? What aspects of your private self are you willing to share? How is your public self different from your private self? What kinds of things have you never shared with anyone?

In a long-term relationship, the capacity to share increases over time. In the next chapter, we will explore some other important self-care skills to help promote self-esteem and reduce stress.

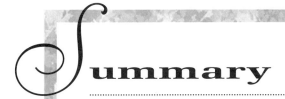

Summary

The practice of positive self-talk is the key to positive self-esteem. Negative affirmations may be old, familiar beliefs, but they are self-defeating. Negative affirmations or self-talk can be turned into positive self-talk. Positive people play positive messages to themselves. Self-disclosure can be used appropriately by the nurse to improve the nurse-patient relationship.

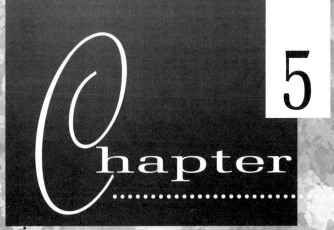

Chapter 5

Self-Care

There is no single way to view life. We all know that life provides neither guarantees nor answers to the staggering problems that face the world. And nurses must confront the additional problems that face the health care system. Certainly, nurses need to develop a sense of perspective, a commitment to nursing, and a meaningful way to view the world in order to survive.

We can choose to view the world through rose-colored glasses. We must work at becoming optimists by engaging in self-care survival skills such as positive self-communication. By talking to yourself, you become more in touch with your values, feelings, beliefs, dreams, and aspirations.

It's important to learn self-care survival skills early in a nursing career to maintain mental health and well-being. Techniques that increase self-esteem and reduce stress are key factors in surviving a career in nursing. When nurses use these techniques, they are choosing growth over stagnation.

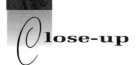

lose-up

The Little Engine That Couldn't

Janet was a first year nursing student in a large urban university. She was very frightened being away from home and in the big city for the first time in her life. She entered biology class with fear and trepidation. She began to think, "They all look smarter than me. I'm probably going to make a fool of myself. I should never have enrolled."

ANALYSIS

Janet is an example of a person with low self-esteem. She is talking negatively to herself based on her past self-images. Janet needs to learn to replace these negative messages with positive ones: "I'm really excited about starting this class! It will be fun meeting and talking with new people. I know I will learn a lot."

Our thoughts are made up of both positive and negative messages about ourselves. These thoughts are influenced by silent assumptions or a personal belief system. A person's belief system is actually his or her philosophy of life. What is your philosophy of life? In order to determine your philosophy, you need to study the positive and negative messages you send yourself.

SELF-ESTEEM: KNOW THYSELF

An important key to finding happiness in life is through knowing yourself. Recognizing your own personal worth is what it means to have self-esteem. To have healthy self-esteem, you must appreciate and value your special talents and abilities and realize the importance of your uniqueness.

To say, "I am a valuable person!" is to experience positive self-esteem. But if you say to yourself, "I'm not important," you are experiencing low self-esteem. We can fluctuate between positive and negative self-esteem. When we feel vulnerable or hurt, our self-esteem can and will suffer. Self-esteem is involved with almost every emotional response and is connected to our individual thoughts.

If negative assumptions are firmly integrated in our belief system, our mental health can be harmed. These assumptions can make us feel vulnerable and prone to anxiety and even depression.

There are many expressive techniques that nurses can use to help preserve their mental health. These enable the achievement of self-acceptance and foster positive self-esteem. Many techniques are described in professional literature and popular self-help books. People with high self-esteem rely on their own judgment and personal values. They set goals that are personally meaningful to them, and they expect more of themselves and strive to meet their expectations. They also take risks and are not afraid to act on their own behalf.

xercise

Evaluating your own self-esteem

1. Choose a specific situation in which you experience low self-esteem.

2. Describe the situation in detail.

3. Identify the feelings you have when the situation occurs.

4. What are the thoughts that go through your head?

5. What do you gain from thinking this way?

6. What do you lose from thinking this way?

7. Can you identify any distortions in your thinking?

8. List some rational thoughts that could replace these self-defeating feelings.

VISUALIZATIONS

Throughout our lives, we hold images of ourselves that color our feelings. Images can be used to improve self-esteem and our sense of well-being. Negative images precipitate anxiety, depression, and a lack of confidence. Positive imagery or visualization is a very powerful tool that can be used for ourselves and for patients. Practicing visualizations can help us to call up specific mental images whenever we want them. These new images are powerful tools for helping to improve our self-esteem.

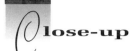

lose-up

Angela's Visualization

Angela needed to take an emergency vacation for mental health purposes. She needed time away from the psychiatric unit on which she was employed. Three suicides had occurred in one week and Angela felt tired and helpless. In order to convince her supervisor to grant her this vacation, she tried the following visualization before entering the office.

Angela pictured herself dressed in her favorite vacation sportswear, wearing her sunglasses and a large straw hat. She had a great suntan and looked extremely relaxed. She then pictured her supervisor sitting behind her desk leaning on a large pile of papers. The supervisor looked tired and old; she was very nervous and fatigued and would agree to anything that Angela asked. Angela pictured herself standing before the supervisor looking confident, strong, and relaxed. She quietly giggled and congratulated herself for being so strong.

ANALYSIS

This visualization was an important exercise in assertiveness training for Angela. By using this technique, Angela was able to strengthen herself in order to request the much needed vacation.

Visualizations are like behavioral rehearsals. You place yourself in a relaxed state, then imagine a dreaded event. By coupling relaxation instead of anxiety with the event, you can eliminate your fear of it. Visualizations can be useful for test anxiety, fear of public speaking, or nursing situations that are extremely stressful. They are also very useful to share with patients.

How to Do a Visualization

Putting visualization to use is not difficult. You can rehearse for a future event by creating mental images of the event before it happens. Since you wish to be successful, you should picture the event occurring with great achievement on your part.

First, you must relax and clear your head of the day's clutter. When you are relaxed, your mind is open to fresh, new ideas. Next, close your eyes and listen to yourself breathe. Concentrate on the air coming in and going out of your lungs. As your lungs empty, take a deep breath.

Repeat the breath, and then take five more. With every deep breath, you can feel yourself relaxing.

Now think about a very pleasant event in your life. It does not matter what event you choose as long as it was a happy time for you. Get in touch with that moment and how good you felt at that time. Begin gradually to think about what you would like to achieve in the upcoming event. Make the experience as detailed and real as you can, from beginning to end. Be sure to make the ending a happy and successful one for yourself. You are looking good! You have just completed a visualization.

Short visualizations can be done quickly, while you are in the process of going through your workday. You can do a visualization in 2 minutes by doing the following: Breathe deeply and slowly for 1 minute, and then follow with another minute of slow breathing while you picture yourself performing with great confidence. Mental rehearsals can provide a tremendous boost to your life!

WRITING AFFIRMATIONS

It is important to identify the core issues related to your self-esteem, and it is particularly effective when put in writing. Writing provides you with an opportunity to address a core issue and its healing affirmation.

My core issue _____

Affirmation _____

Repeat the affirmation to yourself throughout the day. Write it down, and post it where you will see it each day. You can rid yourself of negative affirmations by writing the positive affirmation several times in the left column of a piece of paper, and then in the right column, record any negative thoughts you have each time you say your affirmation.

Here is an example of how this technique works with the affirmation "I can do a great job!"

Affirmation	**Negative Thought**
I can do a great job.	I make a lot of mistakes.
I can do a great job.	I am a failure.
I can do a great job.	I am afraid of success.
I can do a great job.	I feel stupid.
I can do a great job.	I can't do it.

This technique helps clear away any negative thoughts that may come up when you are practicing the positive affirmation. You should use one affirmation until the good you are seeking is achieved. You can always return to it when you feel the need. For the best results, it is important to work with only one or two affirmations at a time. Be patient. Over time, your positive affirmations will help you change your inner reality and transform your life.

JOURNALS

We have all met people who have a wonderful sense of who they are and where they are going. No doubt these kinds of people engage in self-talk, either through mental or written exercises.

When I met my husband over twenty years ago, he was keeping a journal on his life, which included notations on his feelings and reactions. He is now able to review these journals to compare and contrast how he felt about specific issues then and now. It has proven to be an extremely valuable resource.

A journal is a self-clarification tool that delineates the underlying values and goals you wish to achieve. It can be used to record your affirmations and keep track of your progress over time. It also gives you the foundation to make decisions, take risks, and reach your goals. The ultimate value of a journal is to assist a person in determining his potential as a human being.

Journals can be extremely helpful in managing stress and in promoting positive mental health. The writing process is similar to writing nurses' notes. The journal note is a simple logging of events, which promotes in-depth, self-guided personal exploration. The goal of keeping a journal is to identify, on paper, our thoughts and feelings. Writing down our images and feelings enhances our ability to sort out what we find meaningful. It helps us to gain perspective on behavior changes that we are trying to make. Since it is private, we can be totally honest with ourselves. Writing also suggests a permanence through which the commitment for change is enhanced.

Journal writing can be combined with music to help us relax. The music helps slow us down so that images and emotions that are held deep inside can come to the surface. Dating the entries is important because you may want to refer to them periodically. You can track specific feelings and images over time and note when new attitudes and behaviors appear. Positive affirmation exercises can be done periodically to assist in determining thoughts and feelings. Since keeping a journal can be time-consuming, it is a wonderful activity to combine with these exercises.

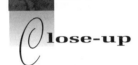

lose-up

Excerpt from Nancy's Journal

June 15th

I find myself feeling as if I can do a much better job now. I've been practicing nursing for one year and I know the ropes. I feel as if I am ready to climb the ladder. For months, I have felt as if I were crawling on the ground. My knees are tired from crawling. It is time that I stood up and walked.

June 24th

Today, I walked for the first time. It felt wonderful. I felt as if I was on a cloud. Everything went perfectly today. I made no mistakes and my patients were satisfied with my care. I can give excellent care. I am a good nurse!

ANALYSIS

It is apparent from Nancy's journal entries that she was working with a specific affirmation—I am a good nurse! The journal entries contain the negative thoughts that she was battling. Eventually, the negative thoughts disappeared, leaving only the positive affirmation. Try a journal exercise for at least one month. It will make a difference in your self-esteem, and it is certainly worth a try.

How to Keep a Journal

Choose a selection of relaxing music and a quiet place. Before writing, make sure you are focused and relaxed. Spend approximately 20 minutes writing about one aspect of your life. Go with the flow of your thought pattern, and do not worry about what you are writing. Just let your pen glide across the paper, recording the images that come to mind. Flow with the music as much as possible while letting go of physical tension. Do not concern yourself with spelling, grammar, or handwriting. You may find yourself writing the same thought over and over again until a new thought comes to mind. Soon you will be able to capture abstract thoughts and make them concrete.

SPIRITUAL WELL-BEING

It is important to note that spiritual well-being does not mean religiousness. It encompasses a sense of inner peace, compassion for others, and a reverence for life. Often, people who struggle with incredible ordeals attribute their survival to their spiritual strength. There are many exercises the nurse can perform that both reduce stress and promote spiritual well-being.

Εxercise

Spiritual Checklist

Put a checkmark next to the activities you performed in the past week:

YES NO

___ ___   1. Shared 10 minutes talking with a child about a common interest.

___ ___   2. Attended a regular church, synagogue, or religious service.

___ ___   3. Helped someone less fortunate than you.

___ ___   4. Prayed for someone.

___ ___   5. Took a walk in the park or woods with someone you love.

___ ___   6. Went to a special church, synagogue, or religious service (or served on a special church committee, program, or related service).

___ ___   7. Read the Bible or other inspirational or devotional material.

___ ___   8. Watched the sun rise (or set).

___ ___   9. Spent 15 to 30 minutes meditating, praying, pondering, or reflecting on your purpose in life.

___ ___ 10. Attended an art exhibit, a theater or dance performance, or a concert featuring religious work (or listened to an uplifting radio program or recording).

___ ___   TOTAL

After computing your total number of yes answers, use the following chart to interpret your score:

Score	Interpretation
8-10	You are probably enjoying all the benefits of a spiritually rich life.
6-8	You have good emphasis on spiritual values in your life.
4-6	Spiritual concerns are a part of your life, but you may wish to spend more time on them.
0-4	Your spiritual life is underdeveloped. Try to bring more of these values into your life even if it takes some effort.

There are many aspects of spiritual well-being that bring the nurse in communication with a higher power. In order to strengthen your spiritual well-being, the following suggestions may be useful:

1. Seek purpose and meaning in life. Look for opportunities to increase your spiritual dimension. Discuss values and ethical issues with family, friends, and co-workers. Pursue truth. Nurture your faith.

2. Take time for centering. Open yourself to the message of a "higher power." Study the Bible or other spiritual or devotional materials. Meditate. Pray. Give thanks. Find time for solitude and silence each day.

3. Make worship or other spiritual rituals a top priority. Prepare with quiet reflection. Participate with enthusiasm. Celebrate.

4. Activate your sense of wonder. Listen to inspiring music. Explore nature—even in the city. Use all your senses to notice the miracles of creation around you. Take time off to enjoy them!

5. Cultivate an attitude of compassion and giving. Reach out, and let your love flow in small and large ways. Listen. Forgive. Respond to the needs you see. Make financial or time commitments to a worthy cause. Help someone who is in pain or having difficulty. Look for opportunities to act out justice.

Promoting relaxation and reducing stress are important for the nurse who wishes to get in touch with the "self." More importantly, visualizations and affirmations help create positive images that assist in becoming that "ideal self." Reaching realistic goals and aspirations in our professional work is necessary in order for us to feel job satisfaction. Our self-images affect how we live and work and how we set goals for the future.

Summary

Self-care survival skills are important to surviving in a nursing career. The nurse should develop and maintain healthy self-esteem. Mental rehearsals or visualizations can assist in strengthening self-esteem. Positive affirmations can help in changing one's inner reality. A journal can be a valuable resource to record affirmations and keep a record of one's values and goals. Spiritual well-being can assist the nurse in communicating with a higher power. Stress reduction and relaxation help the nurse get in touch with the "self," and positive images assist in reaching the "ideal self."

Therapeutic Use of Self, Empathy, and Trust

In Chapter 5, we discussed self-esteem and touched on the concept of self. There are actually three separate images of self: the real, the actual, and the idealized self.

The *real self* consists of the ideas and feelings that we have about ourselves. This is the part of the self that we see when we perform an honest evaluation of ourselves. It contains our strengths, weaknesses, talents, and faults.

The *actual self* is a composite of our life experiences. It also includes our perceptions of these experiences and the images we have of how others see us.

The *ideal self* is what we wish to become. It is the image of ourselves having reached our goals and aspirations in a particular aspect of our lives. Developing a realistic ideal self counter's depressing feelings about ourselves. By controlling negative thoughts and enhancing our sense of power, we can truly enjoy our lives and our work.

KNOWING THE PATIENT

Knowing as much as possible about the patient has always been an important part of nursing practice. Nurses get to know patients by collecting information and learning about them as persons. To accomplish this, nurses must learn to utilize strategic communication and demonstrate interpersonal competence. Nurses must make inferences about patients from their personality, their behavior, the causes and motivations of their actions, their emotional state, and their expectations. Knowing the patient is extremely important when attempting to implement nursing interventions.

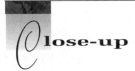

Close-up

Timing is Everything

Jane was a nurse on a 42-bed medical-surgical unit. On this particular morning, she was assigned to care for Mr. P., a 42-year-old male newly diagnosed with diabetes mellitus. Dr. Peters wrote an order for Mr. P. to be discharged in the morning, and Jane proceeded to check the nursing care plan to identify what was left to complete in his discharge planning. Once she did this, Jane discovered that Mr. P. still had not injected himself, so she made that a priority in his care.

Jane approached Mr. P. with optimism. She entered his room with a prepared syringe. Handing the syringe to Mr. P., she asked him to inject himself. Mr. P. threw the syringe on the floor and shouted, "Doesn't anybody around here know what they're doing?"

ANALYSIS

Jane was a victim of poor timing. She failed to identify the patient's status in accepting his diagnosis. If she had tried to put herself in his place, Jane would have realized how difficult it was for Mr. P. to adjust to his diabetes. He was not ready to inject himself because he had not yet worked through his feelings concerning his new disease.

There are a number of behaviors that nurses employ to get to know their patients. Three very important skills that nurses use everyday are the use of self, empathy, and trust. Without these skills, a nurse's work is extremely difficult. The delivery of care is impeded by the inability of the nurse to utilize these skills when interacting with patients.

THERAPEUTIC USE OF SELF

One of the reasons that people choose a career in nursing is that they wish to help other people. Helping others is a normal and frequent occurrence during the nurse's workday.

The helping relationship between the nurse and the patient is very unique. It is a therapeutic role in which the nurse interacts with the patient for the purpose of benefiting the patient in some way. But in order for the nurse to employ the therapeutic use of self, interactions must be structured in such a way that patients are able to verbalize their feelings.

It is important to stress that socializing with the patient solely to pass time is not the essence of the therapeutic relationship. The true therapeutic relationship is one in which the nurse socializes to get to know the patient in order to obtain or share information. A trusting relationship is thus established in which the patient feels free to express feelings. The patient's needs are the central focus of this relationship; the patient feels important and the nurse feels effective.

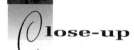

Close-up

Paul's Use of Self

Paul is assigned to care for Mrs. J., who had a stroke three days ago. Dr. Jones wrote an order for the patient to get out of bed today. But Mrs. J. resists Paul. She tells him that she did not plan to be in the hospital with this stroke, and then she begins to review the series of losses she has experienced in the past three years, including the deaths of her husband and sister. She tells Paul that she is too depressed to get out of bed.

Paul listens to Mrs. J. until she finishes her story. Then he tells her how sorry he is for all the losses she has experienced, and that he is also sorry that she suffered a stroke. Paul reminds Mrs. J. that he is here to help. He tells her that he will stay with her as she gets out of bed and into the chair. Mrs. J. smiles and takes Paul's hand.

ANALYSIS

Paul employed a therapeutic use of self in this situation. This was not a dramatic episode in Paul's nursing career, but he was able to use himself effectively and therapeutically in order to reach a goal. He was able to convey confidence and stability to Mrs. J., and he extended himself to care for the patient's physical and psychological needs.

EMPATHY

Empathy is a common term, but a poorly understood concept. It is viewed as one of the most important qualities of the nurse. Empathy is actually the use of several behaviors. It involves the ability to be sensitive to the feelings of others, the ability to explore feelings while expressing sympathetic understanding, and the act of caring in a nurturing way.

Empathy evolves in the relationship of two people over time, when there is self-awareness, positive and nonjudgmental regard, listening skills, and self-confidence. Understanding another's feelings, listening, and displaying a sense of caring are all components of empathy in the nurse-patient relationship.

Empathy is a powerful nonverbal communication skill. The nurse's body language should display close physical proximity, leaning forward with shoulders toward the patient, good eye contact, and arms relaxed and open.

Empathetic nurses are able to appreciate and understand the patient as a unique individual, and the patient feels a greater sense of reassurance and acceptance. This exchange is made possible by the nurse's ability to be truly empathetic. Empathy is not sympathy: The sympathetic nurse is subjective and offers condolences and pity. The empathetic nurse maintains objectivity and offers support and understanding.

It is not necessary to personally experience a particular illness or procedure in order to understand the patient's feelings. But the nurse must be able to communicate the feeling of empathy to the patient. The patient must be able to perceive the nurse's empathetic state in a language compatible with the patient's feeling state.

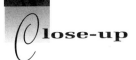

lose-up

Empathy and Sympathy

Bobby was admitted to the pediatric unit with a diagnosis of leukemia. Mary Ann was assigned to his care. She found herself feeling tearful and sorry for Bobby and his family. One day, while giving him a bath, Mary Ann broke down and cried. Bobby's mother was sitting in the room, and she saw Mary Ann wipe her eyes and leave quickly.

ANALYSIS

By sympathizing with Bobby, Mary Ann was unable to be empathetic in providing therapeutic care. If she had been able to place herself in a therapeutic empathy role, she could have even included Bobby's mother in the care. Mary Ann's tears could have been shared with the family. Crying can be appropriate if it fits into the context of the relationship. Sharing tears can be seen as empathetic. Shedding tears is considered more sympathetic.

Why is empathy so important? The empathic nurse is able to establish a more accurate understanding of a patient by tuning in to the patient's frame of reference. Empathy also allows for greater rapport by keeping channels open for patients to express their concerns and feelings. The use of empathy is directly related to client improvement. It increases the patient's ability to cope with serious illness and difficult life situations.

SENSE OF TRUST

Trust is an integral part of the nurse-patient relationship. Without a sense of trust, the nurse-patient interaction would be superficial. Neither the nurse nor the patient would feel any personal involvement.

Trust is the ability to rely on someone without question. It is developed through honest and straightforward communication and requires confidence, dependability, and credibility in the relationship. Trust is also related to the goals of the nurse, goals that must be shared by the patient. The nurse and the patient cooperate to achieve these goals with trust.

A sense of trust is developed over an extended period of time. There are three phases of trust: the orientation phase, the working phase, and the termination phase. Trust gradually develops through each phase in very specific ways.

Orientation Phase

The beginning of a relationship is usually characterized by uncertainty and lack of trust. The orientation phase is an explorative time in which the nurse and the patient clarify their roles. They begin to share personal information in order begin working on their goals.

The formation of trust can be hindered by either the nurse or the patient. The patient is at a tremendous disadvantage in the relationship: The nurse knows much more about the patient, having read the patient's chart and reviewed the reports. Patients who have had negative past relationships with others have difficulty in developing trust. These patients are less able to take risks until they have tested the other person in the interaction. After testing the nurse and determining the safety of the relationship, the patient will begin to trust.

Nurses who have the ability to trust can help the patient develop a sense of trust. At this point, self-disclosure may be useful. By revealing something personal, the nurse can make a meaningful disclosure that allows the patient to know the nurse better, thereby planting the seeds for a trusting relationship.

Working Phase

In the working phase of the trusting relationship, the nurse and patient see each other as individuals, outside their roles. Theirs is a comfortable relationship, with give and take. Both are willing to share their feelings and discuss their concerns. Goals and motivations are shared, and confidentiality is maintained. The patient becomes the focus of the interaction, and his or her inner concerns can be revealed. The nurse may need to use disclosure during this phase to promote the therapeutic relationship.

Termination Phase

This phase marks the end of the therapeutic relationship. If this relationship has been long-term, the patient and nurse must both prepare for termination. A sudden, unannounced departure of the nurse can leave the patient in a state of mistrust. This mistrust can affect future relationships with other nurses.

Student nurses, who have only brief contacts with patients, can have difficulty building a sense of trust. The patient may not wish to share feelings or concerns because of the temporary nature of the relationship. The staffing of ambulatory care clinics, where nurses do not carry the same caseload, can impede the development of trusting relationships. Shortened contacts, in which neither nurse nor patient have had time to develop a sense of trust, are stressful for both parties.

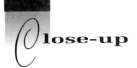

lose-up

Emotional Over-involvement

Maria is a nurse in her mid-twenties. Although she has been practicing nursing for only a few years, she delivers fine care and prides herself on her involvement with her patients. On the oncology unit, Maria was assigned to a 28-year-old patient named Jane. Jane had advanced breast cancer. Maria became very close to Jane, who was recovering from surgery and was now receiving chemotherapy. Maria stayed after her shift ended and spent time with Jane and her family. She visited the family at home, bringing baked goods and other thoughtful gifts.

Maria began to have nightmares about Jane. She also found herself feeling angry toward Jane for needing her so much. Maria finally realized that being overly involved with Jane affected her ability to deliver professional nursing care. She finally requested not to be assigned to Jane and stopped seeing her altogether. Jane was left feeling isolated and abandoned.

ANALYSIS

Maria was overly involved with this patient. This over-involvement caused her to become emotionally drained and overwrought. These relationships usually end with the nurse distancing himself or herself from the patient to prevent further harm.

How does the nurse know when over-involvement is occurring? Nurses demonstrate three behaviors when they are emotionally over-involved. First, the nurse becomes attracted to the patient for a specific reason. For instance, the patient may be the same age as the nurse or may remind the nurse of a loved one. The nurse begins to pay particular attention to this patient and feels drawn to him or her. Eventually, the nurse begins to spend time with this patient before and after work. Special favors are also done for this patient. The nurse gets to know the patient's family, and develops a close relationship with both the patient and the family.

Then, as the relationship grows, the nurse begins to feel conflict between her professional responsibilities and her personal feelings. The nurse feels guilty for spending so much time with this patient and may even feel angry with the patient for being so needy. Finally, the nurse decides to withdraw from the patient. She asks to be switched to another patient and may refuse to discuss the conflict with supervisors and peers. The nurse is left with bad feelings—a mixture of guilt, resentment, shame, and anger—and vows never to get close to a patient again.

BALANCED PROFESSIONAL RELATIONSHIPS

A balanced relationship includes professionalism, empathy, trust, and the therapeutic use of self. As a nurse, you need to be able to recognize the behaviors of over-involvement in yourself, as well as in a co-worker. Assisting a fellow nurse to recognize over-involvement is helpful to both nurse and patient.

Nurses who are over-involved need to take time to assess their feelings toward patients by asking the following questions:

- Does this patient remind you of someone?

- How did this relationship begin?

- How do you feel about this patient now?

All empathetic caregivers get too involved with patients at times. The nurse should be reminded of this and encouraged to work toward a balance in the relationship. The nurse needs to share thoughts and feelings concerning the patient; working through feelings is critical in order to regain professional balance. The nurse could choose to continue working with the patient by restructuring the relationship or by discussing the over-involvement with the patient. For patients who can handle direct conversations, this may be the best approach. Cutting off all contact from the patient, especially if the patient needs that contact, should be avoided. Examples of statements that can be used in dealing with this patient are:

"I have grown very fond of you and your family. You need me to be your nurse more than your friend. I still have very warm feelings toward you and would like to resume being your nurse."

"You remind me of someone special in my personal life. When I'm working with you, I feel very close to you. But in order to be your nurse, I have to begin separating my personal feelings from you so that I can give you the best care."

There is a distinct difference between delivering balanced and effective nursing care and being overly involved. Over-involvement makes the nurse feel tired, angry, and drained. Balanced nursing relationships are filled with empathy, compassion, and a high degree of caring, but the nurse walks away with feelings of satisfaction and a high degree of energy.

Summary

There are three separate images of self: the real, the actual, and the idealized self. The helping relationship between the nurse and the patient is unique. The nurse employs a therapeutic use of self in the professional relationship with the patient. The patient's needs are the focal point of this relationship. Empathy involves the ability to be sensitive to the feelings of others, while exploring these feelings in a caring way. Empathy increases the patient's ability to cope with serious illness. Trust is an integral part of the nurse-patient relationship. A balanced professional relationship includes empathy, trust, and a therapeutic use of self.

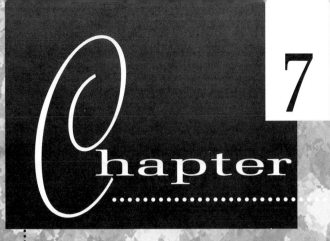

Chapter 7

Active Listening

In this busy world, listening is a lost art. Very few people actually take the time to listen to another person. They are too busy thinking about what they are going to say next. In the world of nursing, how we listen is far more important than what we say. Listening is one of the most important skills used by the nurse. Yet, it is not given the same attention that technical skills receive.

Effective listening increases the nurse's ability to meet patient needs and more accurately address patient concerns. Paying undivided attention to what patients have to say increases our awareness of their feelings, fears, and concerns so that we can provide nursing care for the whole patient.

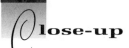 **lose-up**

The Patient Who Didn't Matter

Mr. J. suffered a stroke and was left with expressive aphasia and motor function loss. Peggy was assigned to Mr. J., and he felt as if he was developing a trusting relationship with her. He decided to express his feelings about the stroke and began by saying, "You know, I used to be the number one salesman at Universal Car Sales." Peggy quickly replied, "Oh, you'll soon be back to your old self, you'll see. Many patients have strokes and go on to have normal lives." Mr. J. abruptly stopped talking, and he never mentioned his feelings again to any of the nurses or his family.

ANALYSIS

Peggy did not listen to Mr. J. when he tried to talk about the stroke and how it had changed his life. She was anxious to say the right thing, but chose a response that quickly ended the conversation and made Mr. J. feel that his problem was trivial and happened to a lot of people. In addition, Peggy was not tuned in to the fact that Mr. J. needed to tell his story. Peggy did not need to respond at all—she simply needed to listen.

PURPOSE OF ACTIVE LISTENING

Active listening is the primary source of communication for the nurse. What patients say about themselves is very important. In order to listen, the nurse must be actively engaged in receiving and decoding the messages that patients send. The nurse listens to the patient with two purposes in mind: to comprehend the message and to evaluate its meaning.

The nurse must pay attention to the content of the message, the feelings of the patient, and how the patient states the message. The goal of active listening is to understand the situation as the patient sees it and to translate the message so it can be understood by one's own frame of reference.

ACTIVE LISTENING SKILLS

Nurses who employ active listening are able to paraphrase the message in different ways throughout the conversation. Never assume that you have understood another person's thoughts. Instead, make sure you have received the message wholly, completely, and accurately, especially in very intense conversations. When the topic is emotionally charged or has implications for important decisions that must be made, it is extremely important to confirm the receiver's understanding of the message. How can this be done without repeating the message word for word? It is achieved by having the receiver paraphrase the content of the message. The nurse can simply say, "I think I understand you to say. . . . Is that correct?" Clarifying the content of the message is a vital part of active listening. It also demonstrates to the patient that you were truly listening and the message was received.

The nurse should observe the patient carefully during the interaction. In addition to listening to the content of the message, the nurse should observe body language, eye contact, and nonverbal behavior, and integrate this information to form an impression of the patient's current emotional state.

In addition to empathy and trust, the nurse must use other tools in the one-to-one relationship:

- "I" statements

- Reflection

- Sharing feelings

- Verbal reassurance

- Nonverbal reassurance

"I" Statements

It is important to give patients the opportunity to address their feelings or fears. "I" statements can be used by the nurse to help the patients identify their feelings. For example, when patients are describing their feelings, the nurse can further the interaction by saying, "I hear you saying. . . ."

In situations in which the nurse is having difficulty in understanding the patient's message, the "I" statement "I do not understand you" helps to clarify that the message has not been received. The patient is then given another opportunity to send the message, and the interaction will continue. This response is far better than saying, "You don't make any sense," which will abruptly end the interaction.

Reflection

Reflection is used to obtain emotional responses from patients. Like "I statements," reflection can help patients explore their feelings. The nurse can guide the reflective process by focusing on feelings rather than on information. By saying "You seem anxious," the nurse identifies a feeling that needs to be explored. The patient has been given permission to talk about the anxiety. If the nurse chooses to be reassuring instead of reflective at this moment, the patient's feelings will not be explored. Nurses often use reassurance in an attempt to protect or care for patients. But by allowing patients to talk about their emotional states or fears, the nurse enables communication to continue. Reflection also helps the patient sort out his feelings. It can also assist the patient in not blaming others. When patients reveal their innermost fears, they also feel vulnerable. The nurse must remember to send a message of unconditional positive regard to the patient. With voice tone, body language, and facial expressions, the nurse can convey the message "You're okay" to the patient. This message is extremely important in preserving the patient's dignity and self-worth.

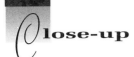

lose-up

Reflection

Ann is a 25-year-old patient with breast cancer, who has been frequently admitted to the hospital for chemotherapy. The staff has gotten to know Ann well and consider her a special patient.

One day, Ann begins to cry when her nurse, John, enters the room. Ann tells John, "I don't think I'll ever get better!" John answers by saying, "You feel as if there is no hope." Ann smiles at John, and they continue the conversation to a deeper level as Ann reveals other fears to John. This nurse-patient relationship deepens.

ANALYSIS

How was it possible to take such a difficult moment and turn it into a therapeutic interaction? In this case, the nurse used reflection in a most appropriate manner. He was able to refrain from using reassurance, which would diminish the moment and minimize the patient's concerns. The patient wanted to discuss the hopelessness of her situation with someone who would listen. Hope is one topic that healthcare professionals often have difficulty discussing. By focusing on the patient's feelings, the nurse allowed the patient to express her concerns and share her pain. The nurse also maintained unconditional positive regard for the patient. All this made it possible for the nurse-patient relationship to deepen and grow.

Sharing Feelings

Expressing feelings by verbalizing them is important for patients, regardless of the setting. In order to understand a patient's feelings, nurses must be in touch with their own feelings. The nurse must be able to both observe and decode a patient's behavior. It is important that the nurse elicit the feelings that are congruent with the patient's behavior.

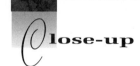

Close-up

The Macho Patient

Mr. W. was on his way to the operating room to have a vascular assess devise inserted for palliative chemotherapy. The decision to have this chemotherapy was a difficult one for Mr. W., and he was very anxious. He took the nurse, Maureen, by the hand and said, laughing, "Everyone up here thinks I'm John Wayne." Maureen realized what Mr. W. was expressing. Macho men do not express their feelings, but in his own way, Mr. W. was saying "I'm really scared." The statement was his way of expressing his feelings of fear and uncertainty concerning his future.

ANALYSIS

The nurse could have joked with Mr. W., and they could have laughed all the way to the operating room. But she understood the feeling being expressed. One way you can improve your ability to relate to a patient's feelings is by putting yourself in the patient's situation. If the nurse was on her way to the operating room for a vascular access devise, she might not have been very scared. But if she had just consented to palliative chemotherapy, she would certainly be uneasy. Sometimes nurses have difficulty in coping with patients' feelings. Instead of helping patients identify their feelings, nurses make incorrect assumptions. That could have easily happened in Mr. W.'s case. The nurse could have misinterpreted his laughter as a sign that he wanted to joke to make light of the situation. But Mr. W.'s facial expression and body language were other indicators that told the nurse that he was anxious and afraid.

Nurses cannot help patients express their feelings if they do not understand their own feelings. Nurses should routinely use some method for identifying their feelings. Keeping a journal, which was described in Chapter 5, is a wonderful tool for identifying difficult feelings. Nurses who do not address their feelings may exhibit side effects such as rationalizing, intellectualizing, and keeping busy.

Verbal Reassurance

Verbal reassurance is another communication skill commonly used by nurses. Nurses often use this skill, but as mentioned before, it should not always be the first skill to employ, since it can and often does lighten a situation. However, verbal reassurance produces a feeling of self-worth and a sense of hope in the patient.

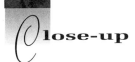

lose-up

Verbal Reassurance

Mrs. P., an 85-year-old patient, is at the point of transfer to a nursing home. Joe, her nurse, comes into her room and initiates a conversation with her to orient her to the nursing home. She tells Joe, "I feel useless and old. Nobody comes to visit me anymore, and nobody cares what happens to me." Joe replies, "I care about you, Mrs. P." Mrs. P. smiles at Joe and takes his hand. She begins to relax and asks Joe to tell her more about the nursing home.

ANALYSIS

The nurse was able to transmit respect and hope to Mrs. P. by using a simple statement like "I care." The nurse can transmit verbal reassurance with simple statements, such as:

"There is hope."

"I am listening."

"I care."

"I understand."

"Recovery takes time."

When the nurse offers verbal reassurance, it must be done in a truthful and genuine way. Otherwise, the reassurance is false and the interaction is no longer therapeutic.

Nonverbal Reassurance

The nurse can also reassure the patient nonverbally through the use of body language, tone of voice, or touch. Some of the most common examples of reassuring body language include smiling, leaning forward, a facial expression of concern, sitting with arms open and legs uncrossed, and good eye contact. All of these behaviors tell the patient that the nurse is open to communicating with the patient.

The use of voice and verbal tone is extremely important in conveying reassurance. Common practices include using a soft tone of voice and a slow and relaxed pace of speech (not rushed), acknowledging patient comments with "um-humm," and allowing patients to finish their thoughts.

Touching patients can reassure and comfort them. The nurse can use a number of gestures, such as touching the shoulder of the patient, shaking the patient's hand, holding the patient's hand during conversation, and even hugging the patient.

Some patients do not liked to be touched. They will usually relay this message to the nurse. It is important to uncover and respect the patient's preferences when using touching as a form of nonverbal reassurance. Although most patients enjoy touching, certain cultures find it offensive. The nurse must experiment with touch until it becomes a natural part of nursing practice, never invasive and uncomfortable.

Patients experiencing lengthy hospitalizations are often deprived of touch. They may tell you that they have not been hugged in weeks. These patients may need to be touched in order to survive hospitalization. The nurse can also suggest soft, huggable toys for patients who experience tactile deprivation. Patients feel more like people when they are treated as such. Busy nurses who have little time to chat with patients can achieve therapeutic moments by using touch.

Tips for Active Listening

Try to remember the following tips during active listening:

- Cut down on distractions. Close the door or pull the curtain and turn off the TV. Attempt to make the room private and quiet.

- Make the patient as comfortable as possible.

- Avoid taking extensive notes, which will distract you from what the patient is saying. Jot down only a few notes if you must, especially statements about feelings made by the patient.

- Sit no more than three feet from the patient to maximize your ability to assess the patient's current state.

- Don't interrupt. Let the patient complete his or her thoughts. If you are rushed, explain to the patient that your time is limited and that you must continue the conversation later. Make a point of returning.

- Use effective eye contact. Be sure to face the patient and show interest.

- Listen objectively by being sure not to show your own personal responses. If you are reacting negatively, you need to explore what makes you feel this way.

- Always clarify what the patient says. Never assume that you understand another person's thoughts. Once you are certain that you understand the message accurately, then validate the message. Active listening is a skill that is learned over a period of years. It is truly an art and takes lots of practice and patience!

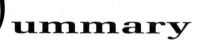

Summary

Active listening is paying undivided attention to the patient with an awareness of his feelings, fears, and concerns in order to provide holistic nursing care. Active listening involves the use of "I" statements, reflection, shared feelings, verbal reassurance, and nonverbal reassurance. Active listening skills are learned through practice over a period of years.

Interviewing Skills

In the initiation phase of the nurse-patient relationship, both the nurse and the patient are learning about one another. The patient will assess the nurse and will be making comparisons to preconceived ideas of what a nurse should be. He also may test the nurse in some way or may even refuse to talk. But as the patient develops trust in the nurse, he will use other behaviors that indicate a comfort level in the relationship. He begins to view the nurse as a person instead of "the nurse," once individual personality traits are revealed.

In the beginning of this relationship, the nurse will need to collect information through the use of a nursing intake form. Such tools certainly help speed up and organize the assessment, but they are often perceived by the patient as rigid and somewhat dehumanizing. Patients often comment on being asked the same questions over and over; they wonder if the health team members actually talk to one another.

USING STANDARD FORMS

Following standard forms too closely can inhibit communication, since they often require just a simple "yes" or "no" answer from the patient. Because of the structure of many forms, much valuable information is lost. Three errors that are perpetuated when nurses use these forms are:

- Failure to listen

- Failure to explore

- Failure to obtain accurate information

Failure to Listen

Failure to listen during the interview occurs when the nurse is unable to place the patient's needs first. By using active listening, the nurse can actively participate in the interview and really hear the patient. Active listening is not used if the nurse is simply reading the questions and requiring simple, one-word answers from the patient. Failure to listen is a gross error in communication.

Failure to Explore

Another error in the interviewing process is the failure to explore. When the nurse fails to probe the patient in order to obtain more information related to a specific problem, the interview is incomplete. Nurses must use therapeutic communication techniques, such as clarification and validation, to further explore patient responses.

Failure to Obtain Accurate Information

Failure to obtain accurate information results when the nurse accepts incomplete or vague answers to questions, without making an attempt to get additional data. When the patient's response is incomplete, the nurse must use open-ended statements like "Tell me more about your pain." The nurse should also explore the patient's interpretation of a particular problem like pain by using open-ended questions to have the patient describe the pain experience. The nurse would need to ask specific questions concerning the location, type, and duration of the pain, and ask the patient to rate the pain intensity by using a scale.

When interviewing a patient, the nurse should choose a private place that is free from noise and distraction.

INFORMATION-GATHERING TECHNIQUES

The interviewing process is a real challenge to the nurse! By using standardized forms, the nurse must be able to obtain all past and present experiences with illness, find out how the patient interprets the present illness, examine cultural considerations, and determine social and occupational roles, growth and development level, and daily living patterns. Techniques used to collect information are:

- Open-ended Questions

- Probing

- Paraphrasing

- Focusing

- Clarification

- Summarizing

Open-ended Questions

When the interview is conducted with a standardized form, the nurse must be able to ask open-ended questions in such a way that the patient is unaware of the structured nature of the interview. This takes talent and experience. Each nurse must develop an individual style, and become flexible enough to deal with patients who have difficulty providing information in a question-and-answer format.

Open-ended questions are designed to give the patient a variety of ways to answer a question. They are extremely useful at the beginning of the interview or when a new problem is introduced. Patients are able to describe the problem, issues, or feelings in their own words and can give as much detail as they wish. This type of questioning is very useful in uncovering unexpected information.

There are many ways to state open-ended questions. The following list provides useful examples for beginning the interview:

Tell me what brings you here today.

What seems to be the problem?

How are you today?

How are you feeling?

Tell me about the accident.

Probing

To probe is to explore in further detail a particular problem or concern. A probe can be in the form of a question or a comment that assists the nurse in gaining more information. The following is a list of common probes:

And. . .

Um-hmmm

How do you feel about that?

Go ahead. Tell me more.

Is there anything you forgot to tell me?

It's okay, you can trust me.

Paraphrasing

Paraphrasing is an important interviewing skill. To paraphrase is to restate the patient's ideas in one's own words. When the nurse restates the meaning of what the patient has said, it gives the patient the opportunity to verify that meaning. It also allows the patient to clarify any misconceptions about the message.

Focusing

Focused questions are opened-ended questions that limit or confine the topic. These types of questions are useful in obtaining detailed information on a particular subject. The following are examples of focused questions:

Tell me about your abdominal pain.

You told your doctor you were nervous. Describe how you feel when you're nervous.

How has your diarrhea been since your last visit?

Clarifying

Clarifying what the patient has told the nurse is an important interviewing technique. When the information received from the patient needs to be accurate, the nurse should ask clarification questions to clearly understand and verify the patient's message.

Interviewing patients can be stressful, especially when the patient is unable to answer questions. Certain questions may be particularly difficult and stressful for the patient. When interviewing, the nurse should always observe the patient's facial expressions and body language for cues. It is sometimes best to leave very technical questions for another time if the patient cannot answer them at that moment.

If the patient is stressed, the nurse should ask clarification questions, with particular attention to empathy, so that the patient perceives concern and interest. The nurse can also teach the patient clarification by demonstrating its use. People are more likely to use communication skills that they observe in their environment. Patients might therefore model the techniques used by the nurse, and learn to communicate more effectively in the health care setting. Examples of clarification questions are:

I'm not sure which medications you are taking.

I'm not sure I understand. Can you tell me about this again?

Could you slow down and repeat that again.

Summarizing

The nurse should make a practice of summarizing the information obtained during the interview, because it is important to review this information along with any feelings that have been identified.

Summarizing is important for piecing together the interview. It demonstrates to the patient that the nurse understood what was said, and gives the patient the opportunity to fill in any missing information. It is also important to end the interview in a way that does not seem rude and abrupt to the patient. The nurse should never simply get up and leave, but should instead use some statement to end the interview. Examples of closing statements are:

Thank you for your help. We must end now.

I must end our interview now. Thank you.

You've been very helpful. Thank you.

SPECIAL INTERVIEWING CHALLENGES

Detecting Discrepancies

Sometimes patients share information and feelings that are inconsistent with their behavior. These discrepancies should be noted by the nurse during the interview. The nurse could explore a discrepancy by responding with a statement that points it out and attempts to resolve it.

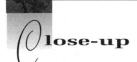

Close-up

Discrepancy

Mrs. P. has been a patient on 2 West for six weeks. She was admitted with abdominal pain and went on to experience a post-surgical infection and septic shock. Whenever the doctor or nurses ask her how she is doing, she always answers, "I'm fine. No use in complaining. There are sicker patients than me on this floor." Jane, her primary nurse, has noticed that Mrs. P. makes these statements while wringing her hands and with an empty look in her eyes. Jane suspects that Mrs. P. is depressed and is using this response to avoid sharing her real feelings.

Jane decides to explore this discrepancy by saying, "Mrs. P., you say you are fine, but your face and hands tell me that you are not. I'm concerned. Would you care to talk about it?"

ANALYSIS

Mrs. P.'s behavior is an example of one of the most common discrepancies in health care—yet one which often goes unexplored by the nurse. Why? The nurse may not want to know about the patient's problem. If it is uncovered that the patient is upset, then something must be done about it. But, by simply talking to the patient about her problem, the nurse is doing something about it. First, the problem is discovered. Second, the patient can express her feelings about it. Then, the nurse can ascertain whether or not the patient requires additional attention, such as counseling or medication. It is important for the nurse to make a note of the patient's feelings. Long-term hospitalization can cause depression, to the point that treatment interventions must be initiated. However, in most cases, providing patients with the opportunity to discuss their feelings is the only intervention necessary.

Obtaining Private Information

Obtaining information on subjects like sexual habits, smoking, drinking, and drug use is often difficult. Some nurses may feel as if they are invading the patient's privacy by asking such sensitive questions. However, these questions are asked within the context of a professional, confidential relationship. The nurse must transmit feelings of empathy and trust if these questions are to be asked with success. Open-ended and clarifying questions work well in obtaining this type of information. Since revealing private information can be stressful for the patient, focusing and probing may also be necessary in order to gain complete and accurate information.

INTERVIEWING ERRORS

There are several mistakes that nurses often make during the interviewing process. Nontherapeutic messages delivered to patients lower their self-esteem and have a negative impact on the level of trust in the nurse-patient relationship.

Leading Statements

Nurses sometimes use leading statements, that is, put words into the patient's mouth by suggesting how the patient should answer the question. The nurse may be making an assumption about the patient that is not true. It is far better to give the patient the opportunity to answer the question without using leading statements. A common leading statement that nurses use is "You're okay," and when the nurse cannot deal with the patient's pain, "It doesn't hurt that much, does it?" Nurses must be careful not to urge an interpretation for the patient, but instead to structure a statement that leads the patient to an honest answer.

Blaming

Blaming occurs when the nurse implies that patients have caused their own health problems. There are certainly many medical problems that are linked to life-style and health habits, but the nurse must always refrain from making judgments. A statement like "Don't you know that cigarettes cause cancer" is very damaging to a patient with lung cancer. When blaming occurs, the patient feels guilty and defensive.

Nurses can identify their tendency to blame patients by analyzing how they communicate with them. Nurses should educate patients by pointing out life-style risk factors that lead to disease, but should always use a positive and respectful way of communicating. The blaming message should be translated into a respectful message, such as "Did you realize that cigarettes are harmful to your health?"

Offering Advice

The interview is not a time to give advice. Nor is offering advice a good idea at any time while practicing nursing. Why? If the patient follows the nurse's advice and something goes wrong, the nurse can be blamed for giving bad advice. It is far better for the nurse to assist the patient by listing options from which to select.

For example, a nurse may wish to advise a patient to take palliative chemotherapy to regress tumor growth. The nurse realizes that this therapy will not cure the patient, but pushes this advice because the nurse likes this patient. Instead of giving direct advice, the nurse should try using a well-structured statement that helps the patient consider the available options. A question like "What are the advantages and disadvantages of each therapy option?" is a better way to help patients make their own decisions.

Remember that when you give advice, you are stating your opinion. You should be far more interested in the patient's opinion. Offering advice during the interviewing process is tempting but should always be avoided.

False Reassurance

Reassurance is often helpful in reducing a patient's anxiety, but false reassurance increases it. When offering reassurance, the nurse must be careful to use it properly and at the correct time. A patient may be feeling depressed and hopeless about her condition. In recognizing this patient's low point, the nurse might actually become uncomfortable about the patient's status and wish to fix things. False reassurance is an ineffective attempt to fix the patient's problem.

Reassuring messages may not match how the patient is feeling. The patient may therefore become more anxious and upset. When the nurse uses reassurance, the motivation should be analyzed. Is a reassuring statement needed by the patient—or by the nurse who may be feeling uncomfortable with the patient's problem? Instead of using a statement like "Everything is going to be all right," the nurse should use a statement like "You seem to be feeling hopeless."

Closed-ended Questions

Although closed-ended questions are useful for obtaining some types of information during the interview, they are not useful when probing or exploring a particular area. For example, if the nurse wishes to know about a patient's use of drugs, the closed-ended question "Do you take any medications?" will generate a "yes" or "no" response. A better probing question is "Tell me about your medications!"

Too Many Questions

The nurse may be tempted to combine questions in the interest of speeding up the interview. This can cause the patient to become confused and anxious. Instead of asking, two or three questions at once, the nurse should break down each question separately. For example, instead of asking, "Tell me about your diet, your sleep habits, and your exercise program," the nurse should ask three separate questions.

Summary

Becoming an expert interviewer takes years of experience and practice. Interviewing is a skill developed by refining the way questions are both structured and delivered. The interview is designed to collect critical data and establish rapport with the patient. By the end of the interview, the nurse and the patient should have established the beginnings of a therapeutic relationship. The nurse should have obtained enough information about the patient to begin nursing care delivery, while the patient should have a clearer understanding of certain health care issues on which the interview has focused.

Chapter 9

Communicating Emotions

The nurse-patient relationship has evolved over the past 150 years. In the days of Florence Nightingale, nurses cared for patients as they suffered with their diseases and injuries. Now, nurses are actively involved in the diagnosis and treatment of human responses.

Today's nurse-patient relationship is a dynamic process between two active participants. Both parties are involved in the interaction, and negotiation is a key factor in decision making. Both the nurse and the patient grow and change. This chapter addresses the communication of emotions that patients experience during illness.

During the maintenance phase of the nurse-patient relationship, the two parties bond, and trust is the glue that holds them together. The patient is moving from illness to wellness, while experiencing a range of emotions such as anger, fear, depression, loneliness, ambivalence, and anxiety. In order to experience self-control and participate in mutual decision making, the nurse must be able to offer therapeutic communication to deal with specific emotions as they appear.

In the acute phase of an illness, the patient is often dependent, passive, anxious, and confused and experiences a loss of identity. The goal of any nurse-patient relationship is to bring balance to the patient's life by promoting independence, activeness, less anxiety, self-acceptance, and self-identity.

THE SICK ROLE

Becoming a patient transforms a person's identity, in that the person feels different or changed. Patients often feel powerless and lose their sense of self. When a patient is hospitalized, the first thing that happens is that his clothes are taken away. Then, the patient receives a room number and a diagnosis. We have all heard patients referred to by their room number or diagnosis, for example, "Please take this to the heart attack in Room 226."

How people are treated when they are patients is extremely important. Nurses need to be aware of the fact that seriously ill people are interacting under a high degree of stress and fear.

PUTTING PATIENTS FIRST

When nurses put patients first, it promotes an environment that fosters wellness and ensures patient satisfaction. Such an environment calms the patient's emotions, reduces stress, and helps the patient to draw upon his own inner resources. By putting the patient first, the nurse is letting the patient know that he is seen as a unique individual with special needs. The use of empathy and compassion are important ingredients for solidifying this nurse-patient relationship.

COURTESY

Courtesy is a therapeutic tool. Simply acknowledging the patient as worthy of attention is a therapeutic intervention. A courteous nursing staff humanizes the environment, making it warm and caring and helping the patient feel welcome. This is very important to remember in a high-tech health care facility, in which a technical environment can make the patient feel cold, intimidated, and deprived of human contact. Courtesy implies respect. A few simple behaviors, such as making a good first impression and maintaining contact through smiling, nodding, and a pleasant tone of voice, transmit courtesy.

First Impressions

The statement "First impressions are lasting impressions" is very true in health care. The first contact that patients have leaves a lasting impression. This impression is created by the first people that meet patients—the security guard, the admissions clerk, the elevator operator, and the nurse who admits them. If patients meet employees who are not friendly and courteous, it will undermine their confidence in the facility and foster negative attitudes and feelings.

Personal Contact

Simply acknowledging patients with a smile or friendly nod can help them feel accepted and welcome. All contacts with a patient, however brief, contribute to that patient's attitude toward a facility. Even if the nurse does not smile, a patient can perceive behavior through body language. Courteous body language can be conveyed through a pleasant tone of voice, comforting physical contact, good eye contact, and pleasant facial expressions. Anticipating a patient's need, recognizing when a patient is confused, and lending a helping hand to a patient who is struggling are also courteous behaviors. Such courtesies sustain and support the therapeutic process.

PATIENT COMPLAINTS

By the time a patient files a complaint, an intense emotional state has been reached. Illness causes stress, but emotions that come from other causes can be triggered. High stress levels begin with anxiety, fear, and feelings of helplessness; the result is often an outburst of anger or depression.

Complaints are most often viewed as problems by the health care staff. But when a patient files a complaint, it is a golden opportunity to turn things around. If the complaint is responded to with a positive attitude, the patient will become a more cooperative and more satisfied consumer.

In responding to a patient's complaint, the nurse should not argue with the patient or become defensive. The issue is not whether the complaint is justified or accurate but how to satisfy the patient and restore his sense of control.

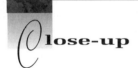

lose-up

The Complaining Patient

Mr. O. is a 65-year-old patient admitted to the hospital for some diagnostic tests to determine the cause of abdominal pain. He is placed in a depressing older wing with outdated beds, dingy floors, and peeling wall paint. Mr. O. is in the end room. He always receives his food tray last, and this makes him feel isolated and ignored. He also is concerned about the results of his tests.

He calls his nurse, Mary, into the room. She comes in and says jokingly, "Mr. O., did they bring you the wrong tray again?" He tells Mary that his food is cold and he did not order this entree. He begins to blame Mary, saying she is stupid and it's her fault that he received someone else's tray. He becomes violent and throws the tray across the room.

ANALYSIS

Mr. O. has reached his stress limit. In addition to feeling scared, he also feels isolated and ignored. Mary should have anticipated that waiting for test results would be stressful for Mr. O. By focusing on the patient's need to express concerns during this "waiting period," this situation could have been avoided. Certainly, a clean, modern environment would have helped, but it does not take the place of a caring, courteous nursing staff.

In addressing Mr. O.'s complaint, the nurse needs to be able to identify the factors that fueled Mr. O.'s anger. By using an empathetic approach and a safe environment, the nurse should allow Mr. O. to express his feelings. The best way to open up a conversation with this type of patient is by saying something like, "I know that waiting for these test results has been hard on you. Maybe you would like to talk about it." This statement lets the patient know that the nurse is aware of the problem—a problem that is more serious than receiving the wrong dinner tray.

No Complaints

When patients do not complain, it may be that they do not trust the staff. They may be intimidated and afraid to let the staff know how they really feel. Or they may feel indifferent or apathetic. They believe communication with the nurse or other staff members has broken down; there is no use complaining for they will not be heard. Some patients fear retaliation. They are feeling extremely vulnerable, and fear that their complaints will cause the staff to become angry and they will become the target of that anger.

It is important to remember that even if patients do not file complaints with the hospital, their concerns are expressed to other people—friends, family, and neighbors. One poorly handled complaint could discourage other people in the community from using the services of the facility.

Important Nursing Behaviors

When dealing with a patient's complaints, remember to:

- Create a safe environment.

- Be empathetic.

- Listen to the complaint. Never interrupt.

- Allow patients to express feelings.

- Identify resources to assist.

- Be objective. Don't be defensive.

Patient representatives are an important resource for nurses dealing with patient complaints. If there is no patient representative, the facility must have someone who is appointed to handle such problems. The nurse can resolve the problem with the help of an objective person.

This third party is not involved in the immediate situation and therefore can function in a calm, systematic manner.

Effective communication skills help satisfy patient complaints and produce positive results. The communication system between the health care provider and the patient should be open and continually functioning. When this system is working effectively, patients and staff experience many benefits, including:

- Reduced stress

- Higher quality of care

- Increased job satisfaction

- Faster recovery

- Patient satisfaction

- Patient energy put into the healing process

- Staff energy put to good use

- Hospital's reputation promoted

EMOTIONAL SUPPORT FOR DIFFICULT PATIENTS

In addition to complaints, several other patient situations arise that demand effective communication skills. Nurses will encounter patients who feel helpless and angry, and who are demanding and controlling.

The Helpless Patient

A sense of helplessness or loss of control often triggers emotional responses in patients. When people become ill and enter the hospital, their normal ability to manage their affairs is greatly diminished. Their self-concept changes, and they no longer feel a sense of control, which can leave patients feeling anxious, fearful, angry, hopeless, or depressed.

The Angry Patient

The nurse will frequently encounter patients who voice complaints about their care or their doctor. While these complaints may reflect genuine health care problems, they often represent anger in disguise. As discussed, most patients will not openly express anger because of a fear of rejection or retaliation by the health care team. They feel weak, helpless, and dependent on doctors and nurses, whom they see as strong and powerful.

When a patient displays anger, the nurse may be tempted to defend the nursing staff, the hospital, and the doctors. However, defensive behavior helps only the nurse and does not address the patient's anger.

As a nurse you may in turn feel angry toward the patient for complaining. If you become angry, you have personalized the complaint. You should immediately stop and pull back. Angry patients are best handled by openness and candor and by remaining cool, consistent, and firm. It is important to stay "in character," in other words, in the role of the nurse. An effective visualization at this moment is to imagine yourself as a tall person and the patient as a small person. Initially, you should also remember to remain standing. If seated when approached by an angry patient, immediately stand up.

The Demanding Patient

Demanding patients are also angry, but their anger is more unconscious and below the surface. Demanding patients desire love and care but go about getting it by making demands. Unfortunately, the nurse's automatic response to the demanding patient is usually avoidance. The nurse may also become angry and label the patient "a pain." The patient's legitimate need for affection and love will be overlooked.

Positive behaviors for dealing with demanding patients involve setting limits and setting them firmly. Within the limits that have been set, the nurse should be available and should show interest in the patient, even initiating contact. The following example illustrates how limit-setting behavior can work.

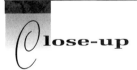

Close-up

The Demanding Patient

Mr. Jones is very demanding, and the staff have become distant and angry with his behavior. He calls for the nurse every 10 to 15 minutes and calls his doctor, both in her office and at home.

Jan, his nurse, has decided to try setting limits with him, in an effort to address his anger. She enters the room and informs Mr. Jones that she is there to talk to him. Jan sits down and makes it clear that Mr. Jones has her undivided attention.

ANALYSIS

During the conversation, Jan is attentive and listens with empathy. She is careful to pay attention to the time, as she has allotted Mr. Jones a time limit. At the end of the time, Jan lets the patient know that she enjoyed talking to him and informs him that she must move on to the next patient. She promises Mr. Jones that she will check back with him within a certain time frame. By using these basic skills, the patient will become less anxious and less demanding.

The Controlling Patient

The controlling patient may be subconsciously angry but does not have angry outbursts. Rather, he struggles to control his care. The controlling patient often challenges his diagnosis and treatment and may even reject the advice of the health care team. In this patient's mind, accepting help may be a sign of weakness, so he instead struggles to maintain control and independence.

Controlling patients are best handled by avoiding direct confrontation. Any procedures and their outcomes should be fully explained to them. It is also imperative to include these patients when choosing treatment options, so that they will have an active role in their care. As a result, these patients will feel less need to exert control over all aspects of their care.

REACTIONS TO ILLNESS

Anger

Anger is a natural response to illness and is to be expected. When patients feel less competent or inadequate, they feel anger at some level of their consciousness. It is important for the nurse to acknowledge this anger, and recognize it as a stage in the patient's response to illness. Statements like "You have a right to be angry" or "I see that you are angry" let the patient know that the nurse is aware of and understands the anger.

Patients with pathologic anger can be very difficult. Such patients have had negative experiences with caregivers. They may view nurses, doctors, and other helpers as people who will take advantage of them. These patients are rather rigid in their beliefs and may be suspicious and self-centered. They will often use the adaptive mechanism of projection.

Patients with a family history of abusive parents or hostile, nonnurturing caregivers may see other caregivers as untrustworthy and dangerous.

In relating to this type of patient, it is important for the nurse to be consistent and authoritative. Bolstering and sustaining this patient's competence and self-esteem will also promote this patient's independence.

Important Nursing Behaviors when Dealing with Anger

1. Show that you understand.

2. Be objective. Do not personalize.

3. Listen without interruption. Let the patient fully express the anger.

4. Keep your voice calm and low-pitched.

5. During the conversation, remain seated and lean forward.

6. Support the patient, without agreeing.

7. Help the patient save face by providing privacy in case of an outburst.

8. Keep an open mind; do not be judgmental.

Extreme cases of pathologic anger are diagnosed as paranoid. These patients demonstrate delusional projections and should be referred for psychiatric consultation. The paranoid patient usually responds well to psychopharmacological and psychotherapeutic interventions.

Anxiety

Anxiety is the most common emotion experienced by patients. It is often the result of frustration, threat, or conflict. The nurse needs to have an understanding of a patient's coping abilities and pay particular attention to how the patient dealt with past problems. The patient's emotional maturity and support systems are also important to note. The nurse must be able to differentiate between normal responses to stress and serious psychological problems.

When a patient receives a depressing diagnosis or responds poorly to treatment, the nurse will most likely note some sort of emotional response. At first, the patient may experience shock or disbelief, and later may become anxious and upset. The patient's ability to concentrate is impaired, but the symptoms normally diminish. The patient feels an overall dread and apprehension concerning illness. Regardless of the cause of anxiety, the physical symptoms are similar. Patients experience difficulty in breathing, a flushed face, sweating, fine tremors of the hands, headaches, and insomnia. A patient can have an anxiety attack, an episode in which the patient becomes extremely anxious, with symptoms such as shortness of breath, tachycardia, and panic.

Medications can be prescribed for anxiety, but there are also several nursing behaviors that are useful in assisting the patient. The interventions vary depending upon the amount of anxiety experienced by the patient. In confronting any patient who seems anxious, the nurse may say, "You seem worried" or "You looked scared." Reassurance coupled with empathetic listening are the primary communication skills needed to assist the patient and to help prevent rationalizations and misconceptions. And in addition to nursing interventions, the patient should be encouraged to seek professional counseling.

Mild Anxiety. Mildly anxious patients are usually restless and irritable. They also have difficulty relaxing in a noisy environment. In fact, the nurse's initial clue that the patient is anxious may be a noise complaint. This recognition of anxiety should serve as a warning sign that things are not going as expected for the patient. The patient will be able to express the complaint or concern in a coherent manner. Mild anxiety is commonly experienced by patients, and it may prove helpful to them in getting the nurse's attention and getting their needs met.

Nursing behaviors for mildly anxious patients are designed to get the patient to focus on what is making them feel anxious. The nurse should take the time to talk to the patient by sitting down and opening the conversation with something like "How are things going?" The patient needs to have time to review the situation by talking about it. The patient may also need validation from the nurse and others that what is being described is a real concern. Supportive and empathetic listening skills are the key behaviors in calming this type of patient. Mildly anxious patients can also benefit from journal writing and relaxation exercises.

Moderate Anxiety. When patients are moderately anxious, their ability to concentrate is impaired. This greatly affects communications, since this patient cannot focus on what is being said. It becomes a problem when directions are being given or when the physician visits and shares information with the patient. A classic example is when the patient tells you that the doctor came in, but he did not understand what the doctor said. Moderate anxiety also may cause the patient to have muscular tension, headaches, sweating, and gastric upset.

Some of the same approaches used for the mildly anxious patient can be used for those with moderate anxiety. In addition, the nurse must direct the patient to try and focus. Empathetic listening is an effective skill, but such a patient would definitely benefit from relaxation exercises or visualizations.

Severe Anxiety. When a patient is severely anxious, both physical and emotional upset are experienced. The patient may have a headache, complain of dizziness, dread, horror, and be extremely fearful. Severely anxious patients have great difficulty focusing and thinking clearly. Decision making is also impaired. These types of patients are unable to understand complex information or directions. They can only receive simple messages.

Successful behaviors for severe anxiety are empathetic listening and quietly sitting with the patient. It is important for the nurse to stay with the patient, even if the patient wishes to take walks or just have a good cry, as the nurse's presence can help relieve some of the anxiety. The patient should receive only simple messages and directions and should not be asked to make any major decisions during this time.

Panic. During a panic attack, a patient is unable to communicate or behave normally. The patient experiences a loss of control and is severely incapacitated in making judgments and thinking clearly. Physical symptoms such as tachycardia, sweating, extreme restlessness, and shortness of breath may accompany the attack. The patient will possibly try to escape from the situation.

Patients with acute anxiety are often brought into emergency rooms. Sometimes, patients experience claustrophobia or agoraphobia during diagnostic tests or treatments. They may express the fear of leaving a familiar, safe place or some other unrealistic fear. It is also possible for patients to experience "flashbacks" of past traumatic events. The anxiety component of post-traumatic stress disorder may be activated in a patient who has had a close encounter with death or has been in an accident or a natural disaster. Patients with a history of abuse may experience vivid memories of painful past events.

Useful nursing behaviors focus on calming the patient by staying in close proximity during a panic attack. It is important to speak slowly and calmly to the patient. The patient should not be expected to listen to complex information or make any major decisions in this impaired state. Deep breathing and relaxation exercises are useful in calming the patient as well as providing a quiet environment in an area away from noise and traffic.

Important Nursing Behaviors when Dealing with Anxious Patients

1. Maintain a quiet, calm environment.

2. Listen empathetically.

3. Offer reassurance.

4. Suggest relaxation exercises or journal writing.

5. Keep messages simple.

6. Suggest professional counseling.

7. Postpone giving complex information.

8. Delay making important decisions.

Anxiety is the most common interference of communication, but it is one of the responses to illness most easily dealt with. When the nurse has a better understanding of the role of anxiety in homeostasis, recognizing symptoms and applying positive interventions can follow with ease.

Depression

It is important to recognize depression in medically ill patients and intervene. Because the medical community has a widespread belief that it is normal for patients to be depressed, these patients often go undiagnosed and untreated. It is realistic to expect medically ill patients to experience one or more symptoms of depression, but not all medically ill patients warrant a diagnosis of a major depressive episode. Addressing depression in medically ill patients can easily be managed in the plan of care.

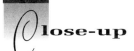

lose-up

Depression

Mrs. B. is a 46-year-old insulin-dependent diabetic admitted to a medical-surgical unit with an infected foot. The foot wound is not healing, and her physician is considering an amputation. Mrs. B.'s husband has not visited her since her admission one week ago. While Pam, her nurse, is making her bed, Mrs. B. begins to cry. Pam says, "Mrs. B., what's the matter?" Mrs. B. responds by saying, "I'm okay." But she continues to sob.

ANALYSIS

Instead of asking the patient what was wrong, Pam should have assessed the situation as reactive depression and said something like, "Mrs. B., you seem depressed." This response gives the patient the opportunity to talk about her feelings. Mrs. B. must be feeling fearful and abandoned. Because her husband is not an active support for her, she must depend on the nursing staff. By talking about her feelings, she will then be more receptive and can prepare herself to accept new problems related to her diabetes.

Sometimes, patients like Mrs. B. are simply given tranquilizers for depression. Although communicating with depressed patients is sometimes uncomfortable, it should not be avoided. Substituting medications for communication is a grave mistake with the depressed patient. Another error is giving false reassurance like "Everything's going to be all right" or "This too will pass." Pat statements like these can increase the patient's sense of depression and isolation.

Mourning Losses. Mourning is a healthy, normal response to loss. Examples of losses are the death of a loved one, the loss of a limb, or the loss of a way of life because of a crippling disease. Other types of losses can be related to loss of self-esteem, such as a role or job loss. Unresolved grief over a loss can evolve into a clinical depression.

The first response to a loss is disbelief. For example, a patient who is told that she has cancer may say, "This isn't real" or "This is like a nightmare."

The next phase is one of anger, as the patient begins to express her reaction to the injustice of having to suffer pain and loss. Sometimes, patients blame others, such as the doctors and the nurses, for their problems. It is important to recognize this anger and blaming as a natural response pattern. The nurse should acknowledge the patient's anger in response to the loss. This will facilitate the development of the mourning process, and the patient will move on to grief.

During the grief phase, the patient fully experiences the emotional impact of the loss. The grieving process involves sadness, tears, and preoccupation with the loss. The more complete the grieving process, the better the recovery. When patients get "stuck" in this phase, they develop a pathologic depression. Sometimes, the resolution of a loss is not allowed to take place. Many cultures recognize the psychological need for grieving and have socially acceptable rituals to express emotions. Some cultures stress bravery and self-control, which can often have negative psychological consequences.

The reintegration phase leaves the mourner with a willingness to accept and enjoy life once again. The mourning period may last from a few months to as long as one year, although the depression may reoccur on the anniversary of a loss.

Reactive Depression. Secondary depressions often accompany medical illnesses. Reactive depressions are associated with symptoms like fatigue, anxiety, loss of appetite, weight loss, feelings of inadequacy, and loss of interest.

Patients may also have feelings of worthlessness, guilt, and hopelessness. However, they continue to function in a "just getting by" fashion. Reactive depressions may be the result of an unresolved psychological response to a loss. Patients who turn their anger inward may also go on to experience reactive depressions. More commonly, reactive depressions occur as a response to illness.

Primary Depressive Disorders. Primary depressive disorders do not have the same etiology as reactive depression. The result of lowered catecholamines, this type of depression is endogenous or primary, and is among the most common of the major psychiatric disorders. Although communication is an important component in treating primary depressions, a psychiatric evaluation must be ordered.

Evaluation for Risk of Suicide. Depressed patients need to be assessed for risk of suicide. Listen to depressed patients for statements like "I'd be better off dead!" or "Life isn't worth living!" Statements like these are messages from patients and should never be taken lightly by the nurse. It is imperative to evaluate the potential for suicide by asking the patient if he is thinking about hurting or killing himself. The nurse should find out whether the patient has a plan or has attempted suicide before. The patient will probably be relieved that someone cares enough about him to ask.

Important Nursing Behaviors when Dealing with Patients Who Are Depressed

1. Allow patients to express their feelings.

2. Sit with patients and take your time.

3. Tell the doctor and other staff when patients are depressed. Document conversations with patients, and that you have informed the doctor of the depression.

4. Evaluate depressed patients for suicide risk.

5. Assist patients in setting short-term attainable goals.

6. Advise patients against making major life decisions.

7. Encourage patients to continue activities that promote self-esteem.

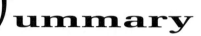ummary

The nurse-patient relationship is a dynamic process between two active participants. A patient's identity is transformed, making him feel powerless with a loss of self-identity. Courtesy and putting patients first are major ingredients in the therapeutic process. Effective communication skills are the basis for producing positive results in satisfying patient complaints.

Difficult patients are a challenge to the nurse. Special techniques are useful in dealing with the helpless patient, the angry patient, the demanding patient, and the controlling patient. Anger is often a natural response to illness. Anxiety is the most common emotion experienced by patients. It is important to be able to recognize depression in medically ill patients. Depressed patients need to be assessed for the risk of suicide.

Chapter 10

Communication Challenges

There are many special communication challenges that require unique nursing behaviors. This chapter will deal with a select group of these challenges, which the nurse will face at some point in the delivery of care. The challenges discussed are difficult because they are emotionally charged and are perceived as stressful by both the nurse and the patient.

CRISIS INTERVENTION

Nurses are frequently confronted with situations that require crisis intervention behaviors. Crisis intervention is a systematic method of dealing with a highly stressful situation, such as a catastrophic death or an unexpected loss. A crisis can also result when a patient is unable to cope with stress that has built up over time. Although crisis intervention requires expert crisis skills, the reality is that nurses must handle crisis situations daily.

What Is a Crisis?

A crisis is a response to an external or internal stress that cannot be managed by a patient's usual coping mechanisms.

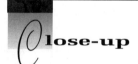

lose-up

Crisis Intervention

Mr. Peters, age 80, has been hospitalized for a fractured hip. He lives alone and has one son who lives in a foreign country. His wife died a year ago, but Mr. Peters talks about her as if she were still alive. Mr. Peters's neighbor visits and tells him that he found his cat lying dead on the street last night. Mr. Peters begins to cry and scream loudly. He is unable to sleep and sits in his bed gazing at the ceiling.

ANALYSIS

Mr. Peters is in a crisis state. He views the loss of his cat as a major life event and has not yet resolved the death of his wife. There are actually, then, two predisposing factors that lead to the crisis. In addition, Mr. Peters does not perceive any resources that can help him deal with the crisis; his son is living out of the country and his wife is dead. He does not yet view the nursing staff as a supportive resource.

Dealing with Crisis

Regardless of the type of crisis, the goal of crisis intervention is to immediately reduce distress, stabilize disorganized emotions, and restore function. The nurse must therefore be able to recognize signs of stress, such as increased anxiety, depression, helplessness, and agitation. Coping mechanisms that are useful to the patient must also be identified.

Effective crisis intervention requires a therapeutic relationship. The nurse must be caring and empathetic when communicating with the patient. While the nurse should be professionally committed to deal with crisis, it may be necessary to refer the patient to a crisis intervention center. Specialized centers are equipped with mental health professionals who can assist in restoring mental health balance with psychotherapy and medication.

Crisis intervention techniques can also prevent a crisis. By recognizing a precipitating event that could lead to a crisis, the nurse can use behaviors to intervene. This technique could have been applied in the case of Mr. Peters and the loss of his cat. For instance, if the nurse was able to intervene when the neighbor arrived with the bad news, the crisis could have been avoided. Positive interventions for Mr. Peters would be built on the therapeutic relationship. Mr. Peters would still experience the loss of his cat; however, he would perceive the nursing staff as a supportive resource. He could turn to this resource as he grieved for his pet. Such intervention is known as bereavement crisis intervention.

The nurse should incorporate the following positive behaviors in crisis intervention:

1. Offer assistance immediately.

2. Identify the problem.

3. Find out if there have been past crises problems.

4. Focus on the here and now.

5. Use problem solving to resolve the crisis.

6. Educate the patient to deal with future crises.

SUICIDE

In Chapter 9, we discussed some initial strategies for dealing with potential suicide. Suicide intervention begins with assessment skills that the nurse can and should use with depressed patients.

Assessment

When the patient begins to give verbal or nonverbal messages that a suicide is being planned or contemplated, the nurse should intervene. When conducting the suicide crisis assessment, the nurse may wish to ask the following questions:

1. Is the patient a male over 35 or elderly?

2. Is the method of suicide easily available to the patient?

3. Has the patient attempted suicide before?

4. Have there been any precipitating events that have occurred, such as the death of a loved one, the loss of a job, a chronic or serious illness, or financial loss?

5. Does the patient have any resources, such as family, friends, and social or community supports such as a church group?

6. Is the patient socially isolated and living alone?

7. Does the patient have a history of emotional disturbances or instability?

8. Is the patient unable to communicate at this time?

9. Does the patient demonstrate hostile behavior?

10. Does the patient have a history of drug abuse or is the patient intoxicated during the assessment?

11. Does the patient display distorted or disorganized thinking?

These questions are designed to uncover the intensity of an immediate and serious danger of suicide. They address risk factors that need to be considered when evaluating the possibility of a suicide occurrence. The more risk factors identified, the greater the risk of suicide.

Suicide Crisis Intervention

Most suicide crises are temporary. The nurse may be tempted to wait for the mental health team to arrive, but intervention must be started immediately and without hesitation. Because of the unique nature of each crisis, there is no set way of handling a crisis to guarantee success.

When dealing with a suicide crisis, the nurse must remain flexible, demonstrate much patience, and adhere to the following behaviors:

1. Make the environment safe and isolate the patient in a quiet, private space.

2. Protect the patient from any family member tension and possible provocation from an undesirable support person.

3. Explain who you are and that you are there to help.

4. Let the patient know that you take the suicide threat seriously.

5. Listen with empathy and care, responding to the patient with verbal statements that validate concerns.

6. Be careful not to argue with the patient.

7. Ask the patient about his plan for suicide.

8. Make the patient comfortable by offering food, drink, cigarettes, or candy.

9. Ask about the patient's problems and what has caused the patient to arrive at suicide as a solution to a problem.

10. Focus on the patient's present problem, considering alternative solutions.

11. Help the patient identify emotional supports, such as close friends, family, and other possible resources.

12. Refer the patient immediately to a protective environment such as a crisis intervention center or hospital.

Behaviors to Avoid

In suicide crisis intervention, there are several behaviors that must be avoided:

1. Never dismiss a suicide threat or challenge the patient to commit suicide.

2. Never tell the patient that he is wrong or make the patient feel ashamed. This type of behavior may push the patient toward attempting suicide.

3. Never try to analyze or interpret the patient's reason for suicide.

4. Do not move too quickly! Helping a suicidal patient takes time!

5. Never take unnecessary risks.

No intervention technique can assure that the patient will not commit suicide. Good techniques and positive behaviors, such as those discussed in this section, can certainly increase the probability of success. But in some cases, patients take their own lives despite the best efforts of the nurse and mental health team.

DEATH AND DYING

It is the threat of death that forces patients, nurses, and all of us to face our own mortality. Every death serves to remind us of the finite nature of human existence. In contrast to other problems we face, death cannot be solved. And we cannot totally prepare for death, since it is something we have never before experienced.

Crisis intervention techniques can help patients who are facing death. For some patients, death is a natural, even welcome, end to a long life. But often death interrupts a patient in what seems like the middle of his life and is seen as a threat to his life's goals. The stages through which a dying person passes, according to Elisabeth Kübler-Ross, are actually common defense mechanisms used to cope with the loss.

The crisis period during the dying process is recognized by its extreme tension. The high anxiety period usually appears well before the death occurs. As patients face the crisis of death, their coping mechanisms either become mobilized or deteriorate and become nonfunctional. Figure 10-1, created from material discussed in *The Experience of Dying* (Pattison, 1977) and *The Deepening Shade* (Sourkes, 1982), illustrates the phases and crises that dying persons face.

Figure 10-1
The Living-Dying Interval

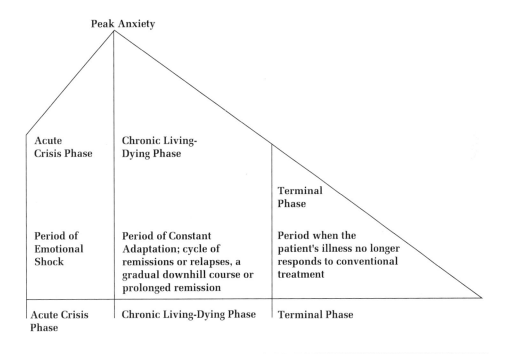

Acute Crisis Phase	Chronic Living-Dying Phase	Terminal Phase
Period of Emotional Shock	Period of Constant Adaptation; cycle of remissions or relapses, a gradual downhill course or prolonged remission	Period when the patient's illness no longer responds to conventional treatment
Acute Crisis Phase	Chronic Living-Dying Phase	Terminal Phase

It is during this crisis period that the patient and his family feel extremely vulnerable. The crisis approach to helping these patients and families cope with death is effective in addressing both social and emotional issues related to loss. Interventions by a nurse who understands can greatly enhance positive coping mechanisms. It is important for nurses to remind themselves of this, for they often feel a sense of failure when dealing with the death of patients.

Communicating with the Dying

Nurses can make a difference in the care of the dying by communicating effectively. Open and honest communication is of primary importance. Empathy, warmth, and genuineness should be combined with "knowledge of self" concerning death in providing the patient a safe place to discuss his feelings. Nurses who work with terminally ill patients must develop their own philosophy of death and dying, because patients can readily perceive a listener's discomfort with the subject. Simply being there for the patient is seen as therapeutic and helpful.

By creating a relaxed, calm environment, the nurse can sit at the patient's bedside to listen, empathize, and understand. Dying patients need to resolve painful and difficult feelings. Feelings of remorse, fear, and guilt over failures in life will cause anxiety. Patients need to discuss their lives and will often perform a "life review," in which they relive their successes as well as their failures.

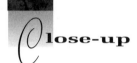

Close-up

Death and Dying

Theresa is a 45-year-old patient with metastatic breast cancer. Recently, she was told by her physician that her chemotherapy is no longer working. Theresa will not speak to the nursing staff. When her nurse reaches out to her, she pulls back and refuses to talk.

When a volunteer comes to visit her, Theresa opens up and begins to talk about her recent divorce. She also shares with the volunteer the statement, "I feel so lonely."

ANALYSIS

It is interesting to note that it was the volunteer that was able to get Theresa to talk to her. Why? What did the volunteer do or say that made Theresa feel comfortable? Patients usually perceive volunteers to be nonthreatening personnel; also, they are not involved with providing treatment and so are viewed as "safe."

It's also important to note that Theresa is mourning her losses. She is not only losing her fight against cancer, but has lost her marriage. During this time she will also mourn her other losses, such as loved ones or lost life opportunities. Finally, Theresa is expressing a fear of abandonment.

Effective Nursing Behaviors

Dying patients need to be able to express and resolve difficult and painful feelings. The nurse can be an active participant in helping the patient only if the nurse takes the time to utilize some of the behaviors that work for these patients. Often, nurses and other health care professionals keep a distance from dying patients because they evoke feelings of sadness and helplessness.

However, the nurse will not feel helpless if positive interventions are applied. The following behaviors are effective for dealing with dying patients:

1. Be present and sit with the patient.

2. Be genuine and open.

3. Give control to the patient.

4. Listen with empathy and give undivided attention.

5. Focus on the patient's agenda.

6. Ask the patient what she has used to cope effectively in the past, to use as a guide for the present situation.

7. Deal with fears of dying, abandonment, pain, and so on.

8. Acknowledge the patient's wishes, asking "what," "when," and "from whom."

9. Acknowledge difficult requests by using negotiation to find reasonable requests that are achievable in the present reality.

10. Maximize the limited time available.

In dealing with the families of dying patients, the following behaviors work well:

1. Encourage communication.

2. Facilitate the sharing of feelings and fears.

3. Respect the individuality of family members, allowing them to deal with the situation in their own ways.

4. Give family members the opportunity and the permission to say good-bye in their own way.

5. Assist the family after the death has occurred, for example, by saying prayers, attending to details of the funeral, helping with post-mortem care, and giving them time to be alone with the dead person.

It is important to remember that long-standing and unresolved family conflicts sometimes arise during this time. Family members are also feeling emotional fatigue, which can cause anger and frustration to be vented at the nursing staff. The nurse can be instrumental in helping the family express their anger in a more appropriate manner.

Family members may also require attention, since they are deeply affected by the death of the loved one. Each member will be affected in a different manner, depending upon personality, relationship with the dying person, previous experience with death, and cultural and religious beliefs. Therefore, it is important for the nurse to encourage grieving and mourning, which helps families deal with the loss. The entire family system must also mourn as a group. Sometimes, individuals who do not have a viable support system need to be referred to a bereavement support group in order to avoid a crisis. The nurse should be familiar with such local groups, as well as with support groups for terminally ill patients. Support groups can serve as a viable support in working through losses, by providing a safe place to express feelings.

COMMUNICATING WITH CHILDREN

In order to facilitate communication with children, the nurse needs background knowledge in normal growth and development. The nurse also needs to develop skills in alternative communication methods such as play therapy in order to communicate in the child's world.

Communicating with infants is very different than communicating with the toddler. Even if the nurse works primarily with adults, the nurse may be faced with the need to communicate with a child.

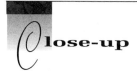

Close-up

Communicating with Children

Mr. M. is a 39-year-old parent with a brain tumor, hospitalized for terminal care. He is conscious and wishes to see his children. Both he and his wife have discussed the matter with the physician and the nursing staff. It is decided that the children should come to say good-bye to their dad. Pam, the nurse on duty, needs to prepare the children before they enter their father's room. She meets the children in the company of their mother to find out their ages and developmental stages, and she will also assess their ability to see their dad.

ANALYSIS

Pam handled this difficult situation well. She took steps to determine the children's developmental stages and used the mother as a resource. However, Mrs. M. is also dealing with the impending death of her husband. She is grieving and may not be able to give the children the assistance they will need in dealing with seeing their dying father.

Pam should seek additional resources at the hospital. The pediatric department may have a child life specialist or pediatric nurse practitioner on staff to assist. Another possible resource is a social worker. Since Pam does not routinely work with children, she may not be able to help children deal with the impending death in relation to their development.

Infants

Communication with infants is primarily nonverbal. When infants are hospitalized, they need to feel a sense of trust in their caregivers. The infant can sense trust through the holding and touch provided by the nurse and parents. Since the infant and parents are emotionally bonded, the nurse must be able to communicate with the parents, who, in turn, translate the messages of the infant.

Preverbal Children

Children who have not yet learned to express themselves through language must be allowed to do so through other means, such as free play, therapeutic play, and art therapy. Through child's play, the nurse can identify a child's fears and concerns as well as strengths and weaknesses. Play provides a nonthreatening way to express feelings and may also be useful with young school-age children.

Children can express their fears related to procedures by using therapeutic play. For example, a child who is going to have a tonsillectomy can be involved in therapeutic play in which she is exposed to the operating room, hospital clothes, and any equipment used that may be frightening. Through therapeutic play, the child's fears can then be identified and addressed.

Nurses who work with children should develop their skills for alternative means of communicating. These skills can be gained through reading, seminars, and through direct work experience with children.

COMMUNICATING WITH THE ELDERLY

Many elderly patients have sensory deficits that can affect one or more communication channels. For example, a patient may be wearing glasses and a hearing aid, or may have an impaired sense of touch.

The majority of elderly patients have at least one chronic disease. In addition, elderly patients are often depressed. They may also be passive, dependent, and anxious. It is important to be sensitive to the communication deficits experienced by the elderly when managing their care.

Hearing-impaired

Hearing loss is common in the elderly. The patient may be hearing-impaired or may not be able to hear high-pitched sounds. When communicating with elderly patients who are hearing-impaired, the nurse should do the following:

1. Eliminate background noise when talking.

2. Speak slowly and in a low tone of voice.

3. Face the patient, allowing the patient to see your lips and facial expressions.

4. Speak in a firm voice without yelling.

It is important to ask patients who have a hearing loss if they have a hearing aid. Sometimes, elderly patients are embarrassed to wear such a device, because they have not yet accepted the loss. The nurse should never stereotype the elderly by treating all elderly patients as if they cannot hear. If the patient tells you, "Don't yell, I can hear you!" you have made a false assumption. It is important to respect the elderly patient; the nurse should, therefore, apologize for yelling and then continue in a normal tone of voice. Maintaining the elderly patient's self-esteem is critical, since, with the onset of age and illness, the elderly patient's self-worth has often decreased.

Visual Loss

It is rare to see an elderly patient without any visual loss. For most elderly patients, prescription glasses take care of the deficit. However, many elderly patients do not readily report a problem with eyesight since they assume that it is simply part of getting old.

When dealing with elderly patients who are visually impaired, the nurse should remember the following tips:

1. Provide adequate lighting.

2. Provide large-print reading materials, especially for patient education materials.

3. Use color coding for medications.

Loss of Sense of Touch

Due to poor circulation, elderly patients often do not respond to changes in temperature. They may also develop foot shuffling as a result of a deteriorating central nervous system. It is important to remember that the elderly have less tactile stimuli because they have less contact with other human beings. They may be hugged less and may not have the opportunity to hold another person's hand. The nurse can address the need for touch by remembering to hold the patient's hand when communicating and by offering hugs routinely. Another way of increasing tactile stimulation is by introducing the elderly patient to soft, cuddly stuffed animals, which can be a comforting substitute in the absence of human touch.

Isolation

The elderly patient is often described as lonely and isolated. In working with the elderly, it is important to consider the following questions:

1. Does the patient have any family contact? How much and how often?

2. Does the patient have a social support system, such as friends, groups, and church affiliations?

3. Is the patient lonely or depressed?

Sometimes, elderly patients treat the nurse as a substitute for a son or daughter. This identification may or may not have a negative effect on the therapeutic relationship. Whether or not such a relationship develops, when structuring communication with the elderly, the nurse should remember to show respect and acceptance and to listen empathetically.

Confusion

Elderly patients may become confused as a result of senile dementia, overmedication, psychological trauma, or depression. In dealing with confused elderly patients, the nurse should keep in mind the following behaviors:

1. Direct the patient to relax and speak slowly.

2. Explain instructions clearly and slowly.

3. Keep statements simple.

4. Respond to the confusion in a calm manner.

5. Be concrete and avoid the abstract.

6. Use all possible channels of communication.

There are many situations that require specific communication skills that can address the patient's concerns. The nurse will be successful by employing the behaviors described in this chapter, as well as by treating the patient as the nurse would like to be treated in the same situation. Empathy is the basis of all nurse-patient relationships; it makes patient interaction therapeutic and positive.

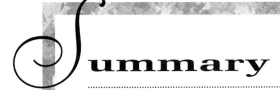

ummary

A crisis can occur whenever a patient experiences a stressful situation that cannot be dealt with rationally. The goal of crisis intervention is to immediately reduce distress, stabilize disorganized emotions, and restore function. Suicide interventions begin with assessment skills performed by the nurse to evaluate this risk in depressed patients. Crisis intervention techniques are useful with dying patients and their families. Nurses can make a significant difference in the care of the dying by using open and honest communication. Many situations require specific communication skills that can be learned by the nurse.

Chapter 11

Families and Other Groups

FAMILIES AND CHRONIC DISEASE

Many chronic diseases begin in youth or middle age and continue through a person's life. Chronic diseases affect approximately 17% of the population in this country, which means that there are thousands of families living with a member who has a chronic disease. Although the disease strikes only the one individual, the entire family system experiences it.

Systems Theory

According to family-systems theory, illness in a family does affect all family members. A long-term illness will generate intense anxiety within the family and alter communication patterns, roles, and boundaries.

The family is considered a system of interdependent, interacting individuals related to one another by birth, marriage, or mutual consent. In order to find out about the composition of a patient's family, the nurse needs to ask the patient to identify the family members.

Communication and cooperation within the family are important in enhancing the ability to cope with a chronic disease, thus reducing family stress. Coping involves two major functions. The first concerns strategies for solving specific problems. In solving these problems, the family reduces anxiety and life becomes more manageable. Examples of problem-solving strategies include identifying a transportation service, hiring a tutor, or getting domestic help. The second has to do with developing strategies to change a family's emotional response to the problems. Examples of these types of strategies are learning relaxation techniques, seeking counseling, joining support groups, and engaging in physical exercise.

In working with families, it is important be able to assess the health of the family. The family system can be classified as healthy and open, or vulnerable and closed.

Healthy Families. If a family is healthy, it will be able to get through a crisis or a chronic disease of a family member while maintaining healthy coping mechanisms. Healthy families are open systems. They have many social relationships outside the family and interact with other social agencies, such as health centers, religious organizations, and schools. These families have direct access to social networks and outside resources from which they receive energy or help (see

Figure 11-1). This enables them to maintain the family's energy to cope with the stressors at hand. These families have permeable boundaries, which allow the family members to have healthy relationships with one another. They also enjoy healthy communication, mutual respect, and a strong structure. These families are receptive to change and have more energy for problem solving and setting goals than closed-system families.

Figure 11-1
Family System

The broken lines indicate the openness of the family system with other systems.

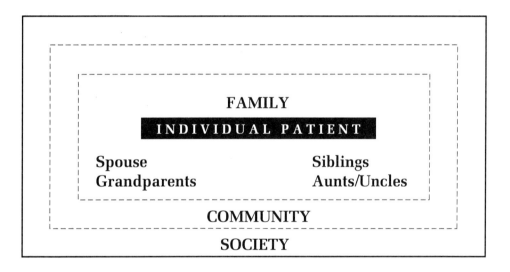

Vulnerable Families. Vulnerable families are closed systems with weak structures. This type of family has restricted networks and little social interaction and does not allow energy to be taken into the family from the outside. In this way, the family is unable to benefit from outside resources. Such families are not receptive to change, and have little respect for family members and poor communication.

These families are highly vulnerable during crisis periods and stressful situations because they have little or no social support. Such families use their energy to maintain tight, close boundaries, which means that the members are highly dependent on one another.

Table 11-1
Differences Between Healthy and Vulnerable Families

Healthy Families	Vulnerable Families
Open system	Closed system
Many social relationships	Few social relationships
Receive energy from outside	Little energy from outside
Strong structure	Weak structure
Access to resources	Limited access to resources
Receptive to change	Resistant to change
Good communications	Poor communications
Respect for family members	Lack of respect for family members

Communicating with Families

Families are complex systems that present a challenge for the nurse. Since the family is the support system for the individual patient, the nurse needs to have the basic skills to communicate with each member. The nurse will need to communicate with the family concerning many patient care issues, such as patient education, home care, emotional support, and treatment options. It is important for nurses to note that chronic diseases such as cancer impact on the family system and affect each family member. Family trees or genograms can be useful in keeping track of family members, noting ages, medical histories, and relationships (see Figure 11-2).

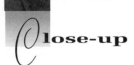

Close-up

Communicating with Families

Lori is 5 years old. When she was 3, she was diagnosed with leukemia. In the past two years, Lori's mother, Kate, has revolved her entire life around the care of Lori. Kate and her husband, Dave, now constantly argue, and their marriage is failing.

Following a recent admission, Lori's nurse came into the room to explain her medications to her mother. Kate could not concentrate on the instructions of the nurse. She stated that she could not give medications to her daughter and could not take her home because the environment was not safe. She disclosed to the nurse that recently she and her husband have had violent arguments.

Figure 11-2
Genogram of Jones Family

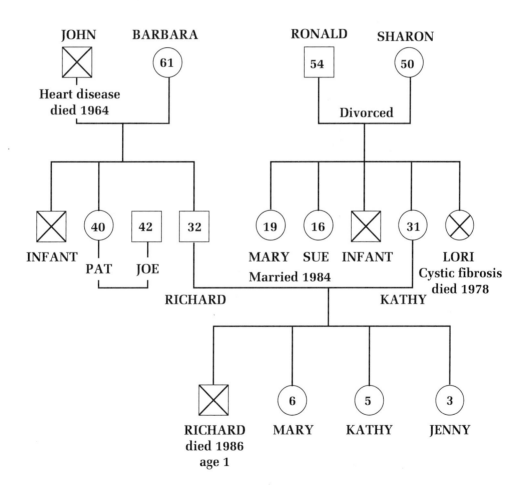

ANALYSIS

In this situation, the nurse needs to assess what is happening within the family. The nurse must take into consideration that Lori's chronic illness has impacted greatly on the family system. Kate, the primary caregiver of Lori, has become emotionally depleted. It is likely that the family is not allowing any outside energy to come into the family system. It is also important to note that the marital relationship is stressed, and therefore the family's positive coping strategies will be extremely diminished. The nurse must work on strengthening coping mechanisms. External coping mechanisms can address problem-solving resources. Internal coping mechanisms can strengthen the emotional status of the couple.

Barriers to Communicating with Families.
Since families are so complex, why would the nurse even bother to communicate with them? There are many reasons to communicate with families. The family is an active part of the care and recovery of the patient. Also, the interaction pattern among family members impacts directly on the physical and mental health of the patient. In addition, communication often becomes distorted when one family member gives information to another that may impact negatively on the patient's care.

Caring for the entire family is a fairly new concept in nursing today. Families have traditionally provided care for their members during illness. With the development of medical technology, the patient care setting has shifted from home to hospital. In the hospital setting, families are deprived of caring for their members. They feel cut off or isolated from their family member and, above all, feel helpless.

The patient's care should therefore include the care of the family, whose responsibility it is to provide love, compassion, protection, and support to their family member. The nursing care will also help improve a family's communication and coping mechanisms.

Effective Nursing Behaviors

There are several guidelines to keep in mind that work well in family interactions:

1. Identify who the relevant family members are and make a record or chart to keep track of their names, ages, relationships, family history, and family structure. A genogram, a kind of family tree, is one way to organize information (see Figure 11-2).

2. Determine who the main contact is in the family, and find out if this person is trusted by the patient. Identify this person's role in the family.

3. Assess the type of family, classifying it as either vulnerable or healthy (see Table 11-1).

4. Identify family members who are supportive and those who are seen as obstacles and block positive interventions.

5. Attempt to communicate with families as a group. Take advantage of the times when families visit, and seize the opportunity to work with the family system.

6. Listen to family members as they express their concerns about the patient.

7. Acknowledge symptoms of stress or burnout in family members. Assist them in developing coping mechanisms.

8. Provide emotional support for families in emotional crisis or distress.

9. Give credit to individual family members and the important role each one plays.

These interventions work well for families both in the hospital and in the home. Being aware of family dynamics and the communication patterns used are critical in order to work effectively with families.

CULTURAL DIFFERENCES

Patients who cannot speak or read in English often present difficulties for the nurse. In many cases, the nurse is unable to communicate with the patient in his native language and an interpreter must be called. If an interpreter is used, the patient should be given time to communicate his emotional as well as his literal response, along with a confirmation that he understood the information transmitted.

If the patient's family members are immigrants, it is important to be able to identify their cultural patterns. There are three types of cultural patterns in immigrant families:

1. Old-time type: This family rejects the new culture and is unable to adapt. This pattern is more typical in older adult immigrants.

2. Assimilative type: The family embraces the new culture and rejects the old culture. This is more common in children and adolescents.

3. Bi-cultural type: The family selectively adopts new customs while maintaining the former ones. This is the healthiest adaptation.

Both the nurse's and the patient's anxiety levels will be extremely high in situations where verbal communication cannot take place. In such situations, the nurse should keep in mind the following points:

1. Identify the patient's ethnic background, noting whether the patient is an immigrant.

2. Find out exactly how much English is spoken by the patient and whether the patient can read English.

3. Speak slowly and identify nonverbal behaviors that can be used to communicate with the patient.

4. Utilize a list of basic words and simple sentences that can be referred to in communicating with the patient.

5. Take time to learn a few words in the patient's language as a sign of respect.

6. Learn the major cultural symbols and traditions of a patient's culture, and show respect for this cultural group.

These behaviors will help prevent the nurse from trying to bridge the communication gap too quickly with verbal interactions. Above all, the nurse should maintain an open attitude and recognize that numerous cultural differences will exist among patients.

Cultural Diversity

Our attitudes, beliefs, values, use of language, and our life experiences are shaped by our cultural backgrounds. Culture is an integral component of the patient's way of life and health; it makes each patient and family unique. Cultural differences are often seen as problems for or obstacles to nursing interventions. But, by appreciating cultural differences and learning to work in a variety of cultural frameworks, the nurse becomes a more effective communicator. The nurse should take the time to identify cultural groups and find ways to improve behaviors that bridge the communication gap. One of the greatest challenges nurses face today is to become more successful in addressing complex nursing care while communicating with diverse cultures and complex family structures.

GROUPS

Nurses interact with many groups. They work with families, support or self-help groups, clubs, organizations, and fellow members of the nursing staff. All groups fulfill certain objectives, since people join them in order to reach a goal. The nature of the goal set by a group determines the type of group and its life span. Task groups are different from therapeutic groups in terms of focus, purpose, techniques used to facilitate group goals, roles and functions of members, and type of membership.

Task Group

A task group is a type of work group. Its focus is getting the job done. Examples of task groups are a nursing staff, a hospital committee, or a softball team. These groups concentrate on the content of the task at hand. A task group's meetings will involve proposing, discussing, making decisions, and evaluating ideas that relate to getting the job done. Members of a task group will make suggestions, give opinions, clarify issues, keep records, summarize content, and plan for future meetings.

The leader of a task group is often selected from within the group. The leader's role differs from the members, in that this person is responsible for guiding the group in deciding its purpose and goals, and uses skills that focus on the process of working together. The leader needs to be aware of ways to utilize the group's total resources. The leader must therefore be able to identify the individual members as resources and objectively assess their strengths and limitations. The leader must also be able to help the group progress toward accomplishing its goals as well as identify alternatives.

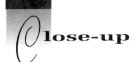

lose-up

Task Group

Ann, a staff nurse on an obstetrics unit, was recently approached by the nursing manager to chair a committee on patient relations for the unit.

Although Ann was a recent graduate, the manager thought that she had great leadership potential, and wanted to give her the opportunity to develop her talents.

Ann formed a unit-based committee by selecting staff nurses to become members and then set up a schedule of meetings. To Ann's disappointment, only one staff nurse attended the meetings. She participated minimally while Ann did all the work. Ann reported to her manager that she was very discouraged and felt the staff did not like her.

ANALYSIS

Ann's problem was not that the staff did not like her. Rather, the staff had not been approached about becoming members of this group and did not have an understanding of its purpose. Ann also did not have any legitimate authority over the staff, and without power, she could not proceed.

Although the nursing manager was willing to support Ann, the members did not. There are a few reasons for their lack of support. First, they may have wanted Ann to fail. Second, they may have been angry with the manager for not selecting one of them to lead the group. Group dynamics play a major part in the success or failure of groups. The dynamics in this situation caused the group to fail. Group communication is similar to other types of communication in that messages are sent to and received by individuals and the group at large (see Figure 11-3).

Group Leader Behaviors. The behavior of the group leader affects the members of the group. There are three major types of leadership styles: autocratic, democratic, and laissez-faire. The autocratic leader is directive and makes decisions for the group. Ann's nursing manager was this type of leader. She never consulted the group for their opinions. The democratic leader involves the group in decision making. The laissez-faire leader has a very loose control over the membership. Ann's leadership style was probably also autocratic; she may have modeled her behavior after her nursing manager. Nurses will often model their behavior after leaders they observe in practice. It is better to develop your own leadership style based on your own personality and the situation. One particular type of leadership style may be more effective, depending upon the task, the structure and size of the group, and the personalities of the members.

Figure 11-3
Group Communication

Messages are sent to and received by individuals and the group.

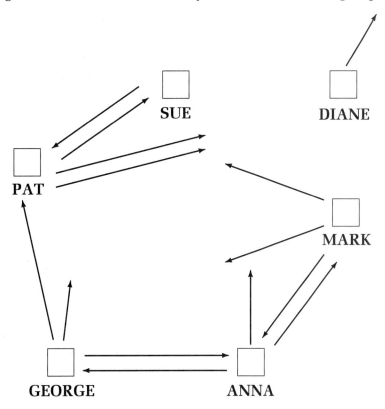

Process Work. All groups do something called process work, which creates and maintains the climate needed to reach group goals. Group dynamics are related to group norms, behaviors, expectations, and the phase of the group. Group dynamics will be discussed in more detail later in this chapter.

Therapeutic Groups

Therapeutic groups also meet for a specific purpose. This purpose is usually related to emotional growth, developing human relationships, or coping with specific problems. Examples of therapeutic groups are

Alcoholics Anonymous, cancer support groups, breastfeeding groups, or bereavement groups. These groups differ in terms of their goals, membership, techniques, and the role of the leader.

Many therapeutic groups address several methods that support growth, including cognitive, behavioral, experiential, and emotional methods. The members are encouraged to look at alternatives and to make choices in developing a better sense of self-control.

The leader of the group needs to be able to model appropriate behavior and to communicate openly with the members in a caring, supportive manner. Empathetic listening is a key skill, as it is important for the leader to demonstrate care and concern for all group members. In addition to active listening, the group leader uses facilitating, clarifying, questioning, supporting, and summarizing. The leader also must be skillful in analyzing situations and synthesizing information. Being flexible and having a sense of humor also helps facilitate a group. In addition, the group leader must have a clear understanding of self.

Self-Help Groups. It is important to note the difference between a self-help group and a support group. A self-help group is a mutual support system aimed at helping people overcome a problem, thereby helping members have a greater sense of self control. The membership structure encourages active participation and individual responsibility. The members also act as role models for one another. By disclosing their personal experiences, the members provide each other with a unique type of support and acceptance.

The leader of a self-help group has experienced the same type of problem as the members. The nurse is not typically the leader, but often assists in organizing and facilitating the first phase of this type of group. The task of leadership is gradually turned over to the members as their comfort level increases.

Support Groups. A support group provides mutual support and a safe atmosphere for people to discuss specific issues common to the group. For instance, a cancer support group would help members increase their knowledge of cancer while dispelling misconceptions. In addition to receiving mutual support, members have the opportunity to make changes in their lives. The group provides a forum in which to discuss these life changes and members' difficult experiences. This type of group is usually socially connected and members are encouraged to phone each other or car pool to meetings. The social network created by the membership is important in that the leader is not seen as the only person on which members can rely.

The leader of a support group is usually a professional and sometimes a nurse. In order to function in this role, the nurse should have a knowledge of the problem experienced by the members; however, it is not necessary to have personally experienced the problem in order to successfully lead this group. Empathetic nurses can lead support groups and be viewed as sincerely interested in the members. The skills of a support group leader are related to educating, supporting, and assisting the members to grow.

Group Issues

Ideally, a group should have a balance between task work and the process and communication needed to get the job done. One major issue concerns the group's struggle for identity. Group identity sets the stage for the identification of acceptable group behaviors.

Sometimes an individual group member's needs cause tension in a group. This member's personal needs may get in the way of the group's agenda, imposing on the group's needs and goals. The individual group member must come to terms with whether or not that group can meet her personal needs.

Another issue in groups is related to power and control. Members must come to terms with the amount of power each has and with which members control the group. There is often an unconscious agreement about the balance of power and which members possess it.

Lastly, the issue of intimacy and trust in groups is critical. As members become more trusting of one another, they will be more inclined to disclose and interact on a personal level. Intimate and trusting groups have a solid frame in which to deal with sensitive emotional issues. The group can also offer a refuge to vulnerable members who need a safe environment in order to deal with crisis or pain.

Phases of Groups

Groups evolve and develop over time. Group dynamics are related to the phase of group development. The tasks chosen and the issues raised also relate to the specific developmental phase of the group.

Preaffiliation. When members first come into a group, they behave according to the standard set by their previous group affiliation. The major concerns of this initial group phase are trust and identity. The members will often maintain a distance from one another. Some members will make excuses to avoid the group yet verbally state that they wish to become members. This ambivalence is accompanied by anxiety.

Effective nursing behaviors for the preaffiliation phase are

1. Active listening

2. Empathy

3. Respect

4. Encouraging shared responsibility

5. Sincerity

Power and Control. In the next phase, the group deals actively with power and control. Issues such as which members have authority and influence and how decisions are made are resolved. There may be aggressive competition among the members for leadership, to the point that they challenge the appointed leader. The group leader needs to encourage the expression of feelings and anxieties during this phase so that the group can move on to the next phase.

Effective nursing behaviors for the power and control phase are

1. Directing

2. Clarifying

3. Questioning

4. Active listening

5. Problem solving

Intimacy. In the intimacy phase, trust and intimacy increase to the level that self-disclosure is more comfortable for the members. There may be conflicts during this phase, since some members may be more dependent on the group than others. Some of these conflicts may be related to relationships and responsibilities. Members may complain about other group members who monopolize or do not participate. Or members may ask too many questions or give too much advice to other members.

Effective nursing behaviors for the intimacy phase are

1. Resolving conflicts

2. Clarifying

3. Problem solving

4. Tactful "gate-closing" to slow down overtalkers

Differentiation. The differentiation phase is the working phase of the group, with trust and commitment evident among the members. The group is able to show caring and mutual support. It has formed its identity, and there is a feeling of cohesion and cooperation. The work of the group gets accomplished through shared responsibility, and conflict is minimal.

Effective nursing behaviors for the differentiation phase are

1. Decision making

2. Self-disclosure

3. Reporting

4. Summarizing

5. Mutual sharing

6. Empowerment

Termination. In the termination phase of the group, there is an opportunity to review and reflect the group's accomplishments. At this time, the anxiety of the members will rise, since leaving the group is emotional. Although some groups go on indefinitely, individual members may leave. The group leader should become very active in this phase, employing strategies that work to ensure positive termination.

Effective nursing behaviors for the termination phase include the following:

1. Summarizing

2. Discussion

3. Active listening

4. Awareness

5. Reflection

6. Evaluation

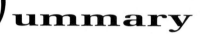ummary

Working with families and groups requires leadership and communication skills. Effective communication skills in group work take experience and practice. Some nurses find working with families and groups to be a bit overwhelming. Nurses who are able to deal with the complexities of a group are able to offer a higher level of nursing skills in diversified health care settings.

Chapter 12

Humor and Spirituality

HUMOR AND HEALTH CARE

A primary goal of nursing is to help patients and families cope with illness or the threat of illness. Humor is one positive coping mechanism that promotes communication. Increasing numbers of nurses are recognizing the benefits of humor in the therapeutic nurse-patient relationship. The need to laugh is as basic as the need for love, security, and safety. Humor is an effective tool for normalizing a terrifying situation and breaking down communication barriers. It is particularly beneficial for patients under stress.

How Humor Works

The relationship between humor and health was first recognized by Norman Cousins in 1964. He wrote about the physiological effects of humor in a book called *Anatomy of an Illness*. He described how specific humor interventions assisted him in recovering from a collagen disease in 1964. Later, he used similar strategies in recovering from a myocardial infarction. Cousins believed that humor freed the body of negative emotions that interfered with the healing process. He also used humor as a technique for neutralizing emotions and restoring hope.

Vera Robinson, considered by some to be the "fairy godmother of humor," identified four functions of humor related to the health of patients:

1. Communication

2. Socialization

3. Psychological function

4. Physiological function

Communication. Humor has a communication function when it helps relay a message that may be emotional or unacceptable. The message is communicated indirectly by using humor to disguise the true message.

For example, a patient is on his way to the operating room. He grabs his nurse's hand and says, "Everybody around here thinks I'm John Wayne!" Then the patient laughs. As the nurse responds, she notices that the patient's face is flushed and dripping with perspiration. His body language says that he is anxious, but his verbal message is light and joking. In order to understand the patient's communication, the nurse must consider both the verbal and nonverbal messages. This patient had great difficulty expressing his true feelings and emotions, but he is able to communicate his feelings through the use of humor. If the nurse chose to simply laugh along with this patient, the true message would have been missed. She also would not be able to be therapeutic at a critical time.

Socialization. Humor also provides a coping mechanism to deal with embarrassing or difficult situations. It assists in establishing nurse-patient relationships by reducing the tension in an unfamiliar environment. When nurses use humor to socialize, they are helping to normalize the situation. A patient may feel uncomfortable about wearing a hospital gown. By making a joke about the hospital's new "designer" gowns, the nurse may help the patient feel less tense and the relationship between the nurse and the patient will grow.

Psychological Function. Humor reduces stress; it provides a means to release tension, anxiety, hostility, and anger. By using humor to adapt to a stressful situation, the patient will feel more relaxed and have a greater sense of well-being. The physiologic and biochemical research conducted on humor is an exciting breakthrough in documenting the healthful properties of laughter.

Humor is sometimes seen as a defense mechanism to help the patient distance himself from a problem. By creating this distance, the patient gains perspective and insight. Humor may be incorporated into stress management classes and other relaxation techniques to decrease anxiety. Humor is thus a coping strategy that has implications for health promotion and the prevention of disease.

Physiological Function. Humor has a definite physiological effect. When someone laughs, the heart rate and blood pressure are initially raised. After the laugh, both the heart rate and the blood pressure drop to a below-normal level. Laughter increases respirations, oxygen saturation levels, muscular activity, and the production of catecholamines, which stimulate the production of endorphins. Norman Cousins first identified the endorphins released by laughter when he was able to get two hours of pain-free sleep after ten minutes of "belly laughing." Humor is a valuable asset to physical health, in preventing disease and in reducing stress.

Humor Assessment

A humor assessment is an important tool for determining the use of humor as a coping intervention for patients. In very high stress situations, such as when a patient receives a serious diagnosis or is told that she is dying, the use of humor is inappropriate. Another situation in which humor would be in bad taste is when a patient has been told that his treatment has failed. Humor interventions become more successful as the stress level drops. When a patient begins to use a sense of humor, the process of healing or recovery has begun.

There are many different ways to perform a humor assessment. The goal of the assessment is to find out what makes the patient smile or laugh.

Some questions that are important to include in a humor assessment are:

1. When you feel sad or tense inside, what helps you relax?

2. When you were a child, what was your favorite toy?

3. Do you have a favorite cartoon character?

4. Who in your family should get the "best giggler" award?

5. Can you recall the funniest movie that you ever saw?

6. Who is your favorite comedian?

Humor Interventions

For caregivers as well as patients, humor activities provide a unique opportunity to relate to each other less seriously and more like children. The stress of disease makes patients feel sad, depressed, and worried. Humor can replace these negative emotions with positive ones. The tense, sad patient becomes relaxed and happy. It is certainly a great stress management technique.

Humor also promotes intimacy between the nurse and the patient. The emotional bond between the two is strengthened through the sharing of humor. The nurse can benefit from humor nearly as much as the patient.

Humor Props

A variety of humor props can be used at the bedside. Many resemble children's toys. Clown noses, funny glasses, bubbles, wind-up toys, silly hats, balloons, and magic tricks are some of the most popular. Props can be kept in a basket or even an old pillowcase to create a humor bag. When patients begin to identify their humor resources, they may select favorites or introduce the nurse to many new ones.

Some patients enjoy listening to their favorite comedian on an audiotape or will ask to see videotapes of contemporary or vintage comedies. Classics like *Who's on First* with Bud Abbott and Lou Costello or Laurel and Hardy's *The Great Pie Fight* are enjoyed by patients of all ages. It is important to think of these films as distractors. Watching light, funny films helps to create the perspective or distance necessary for working through the emotions associated with a serious illness.

Decorating hospital equipment can be a stress-reducer. Putting a bright red wig on the blood pressure machine or hanging decorations on the IV pole helps create a different, nonthreatening image of therapies that the patient might find frightening. Some patients are extremely frightened of chemotherapy and view the IV pole and solution container as "the enemy." By decorating the pole with cheerful stuffed animals or party streamers, this association can be changed.

Humor props promote communication, since visitors and staff will often stop to enjoy them. Humor breaks are created by spreading humor props throughout the clinical area. The nurse is able to identify stressful points for patients, such as before a dreaded treatment or the visit of a difficult relative, and may wish to prescribe a humor break for patients at these times.

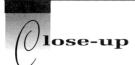

lose-up

Humor Intervention

Mr. Brown is an 80-year-old patient with cancer of the lung and brain metastasis. He attempts to get out of bed constantly, so a chest restraint had to be instituted.

Mr. Brown tries to get out of the restraint and fails. In frustration, he begins to shout to the nursing staff to get him out of the jacket. Phyllis, his nurse, decides that she must intervene. She goes to her humor bag and pulls out a jumbo pair of plastic scissors. She brings them to Mr. Brown and instructs him to use them to cut off the restraint. Mr. Brown takes the scissors from her and begins to laugh. He gives up his fight and begins to relax.

ANALYSIS

Phyllis' humor intervention was successful because it created distance from a serious subject and also worked as a stress reducer during the patient's "fight or flight" attempt. This nurse selected an appropriate humor prop for the situation in order to communicate a message. The patient was able to respond to the message. The nurse felt good about the intervention and shared in the humor. Both the nurse and the patient benefited.

The timing of this intervention was just right, and no one got hurt. Bad timing is when humor is used at an inappropriate moment. This nurse did not laugh at the patient, she laughed with him. Humor should never be used at someone's expense.

Humor for Nurses

Who ever said that being a nurse is not any fun? Nurses need to take their work seriously but themselves lightly. Showing your sense of humor adds to the therapeutic relationship. Laughter creates a bond between the nurse and the patient and reduces stressful events.

Nurses need to use humor interventions for their own benefit. They need to support one another, for example, by taking "laugh breaks." This can be done easily and discretely by going into a nurses lounge or the cafeteria. Using humor props, telling jokes, and practicing belly laughs are just some of the many ways to enjoy humor on the job.

Ways to Enjoy Humor

1. Make a humor bag that contains some of the things that make you laugh.

2. Post something funny in your work area or in the staff bathroom.

3. Create a humor bulletin board, and interest the staff in posting jokes and funny pictures on it.

4. Use humorous calendars.

5. Circulate a spoof memo.

6. Post humor signs.

7. Collect clowns.

8. Send funny cards and gifts.

9. Keep cartoon books and joke books around in the work area to be shared by others.

10. Have a funny hat day.

11. Make a scrapbook containing all your favorite jokes and cartoons.

12. Have a surprise party.

13. Before a staff meeting, share a funny story.

14. Share funny stories about yourself.

15. Use exaggeration to gain perspective.

16. Play a funny audiotape in your car on your way home from work.

17. Watch humorous videotapes, especially after a difficult day.

18. Take a humor break. Smile and take a deep breath.

19. Schedule some time to have fun!

20. Stand back and look for the humor in everyday events.

SPIRITUALITY

Spirituality has a different meaning for every person. Some think of it as a person's spiritual orientation. Others think of it as how a person communicates with a higher power. Many patients turn to spirituality to search for the meaning of life or for answers to why they have a serious or life-threatening illness. Some patients become angry with God because He caused the disease to occur. Others interpret the disease as a part of their spiritual journey.

Nurses may be uncomfortable assisting patients with their spiritual needs, especially if they have not resolved their own feelings about spirituality. In order to be comfortable with patients' spirituality, nurses need to establish their own personal philosophy. Nurses must explore and address their own feelings and attitudes so they are able to assist others. Regardless of their own beliefs, nurses must respect and support the spiritual beliefs of all patients. More important, they should not assume certain beliefs in patients or force beliefs on those who may be agnostics or atheists.

There are several communication tools that become useful in helping patients through these difficult life situations, including visualization, hope, and prayer.

Visualization

Visualization can be used to enhance one's spiritual dimension. Religious visualization might include an image of God or some higher power standing in a garden or on a cloud. The patient may find comfort in the image of God standing there waiting to receive the patient with open arms and a pleasant smile. A patient could also be encouraged to smell the fragrance of the flowers or feel the cloud beneath his feet. Visualization helps patients feel that they will not be left alone, and is especially useful to patients and families facing death.

The nurse can guide the patient through a spiritual visualization by speaking slowly and clearly in describing positive images that reduce anxiety and calm the patient. It is important to find out what images the patient finds helpful.

Hope

Hope is closely related to faith, which is the belief in and reliance on a higher power. Faith can help patients maintain a hopeful attitude even when dealing with difficult illnesses. When patients feel hopeful, they have faith, confidence, and determination. When patients lose faith, they feel despair, hopelessness, doubt, depression, apathy, sadness, and grief. Patients sometimes fluctuate between hope and despair, depending upon their physical state, interpersonal experiences, cultural attitudes, environmental factors, and spiritual beliefs.

The following nursing behaviors support hope:

1. Allow the patient time to talk. Use active listening skills to assist the patient in identifying concerns and expressing feelings.

2. Provide a supportive, hopeful climate in which the patient feels safe.

3. Discuss problem-solving strategies with the patient to identify new coping skills that give the patient a sense of control.

4. Support positive relationships with identified members of the patient's support group.

Prayer

Prayer is communication with a higher power. Although it is often associated with religious institutions, such as a church or synagogue, it can be used anywhere.

The nurse's spiritual interventions may involve either reading the Bible or praying with the patient. However, the nurse may feel uncomfortable in joining in prayer with patients or their families. In such cases, the use of silence shows respect and acceptance. When patients are in great conflict over their spirituality, the nurse should contact the hospital chaplain or the appropriate clergy from the patient's house of worship. The nurse should refrain from debating religious issues with patients and should never preach personal beliefs to patients.

In dealing with a patient's despair, the nurse can be available to share the pain. Prayer can be a source of strength for both the patient and the nurse. It provides the opportunity to express many different feelings. Sometimes anger and disappointment are expressed. For example, in the Thirteenth Psalm, "How much longer will you forget me, Lord?" sounds like a cry of despair. Other prayers provide comfort and express acceptance. While the Thirteenth Psalm expresses depression and loneliness, it ends with the verse "For you will never let me go."

The following behaviors should be used in addressing patient's spiritual concerns:

1. Listen to the patient.

2. Identify the patient's needs or feelings regarding spirituality.

3. Allow the patient to express despair or hope.

4. Respond positively to the patient's requests for prayer. Learn how to pray with your patients.

Communicating with God or a higher power can nourish patients and guide them through illnesses and pain.

SPIRITUALITY AND THE NURSE

Prayer and spirituality are interventions for spiritual healing. Nurses, too, need to have hope and strength. Taking spiritual care of themselves allows nurses to care for the needs of others.

The Serenity Prayer is particularly relevant for nurses.

God grant me the serenity to accept the things I cannot change, the courage to change the things I can, and the wisdom to know the difference.

This prayer is an example of a communication the nurse has with a higher power. Prayer deepens the nurse's spiritual life and provides the strength to continue caring for others.

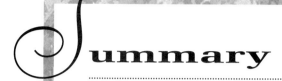

Summary

Humor is a positive coping mechanism that promotes communication. It also reduces stress and helps create perspective in difficult situations. The physiologic effects of humor have been proven through research. Nurses can perform humor assessments in order to find out what makes a patient laugh or smile. Communication tools that enhance one's spirituality are visualization, hope, and prayer.

Public Speaking

Public speaking plays an important role in nursing because it helps to inform the public and deals with professional issues and controversies. To be an effective public speaker, the nurse must have both credibility and the ability to deliver the message.

PROFESSIONAL CREDIBILITY

Professional credibility is based on trust. The audience needs to trust the speaker in order to believe the message. Therefore, the speaker should have a reputation for being not only knowledgeable and informative, but also trustworthy.

The speaker's attitude toward self, the message, and the audience can affect credibility. A nurse's attitude toward himself or herself may be conscious or unconscious. For example, if a nurse feels incompetent or unworthy, it will be evident in the message. We cannot expect others to believe in us if we do not believe in ourselves. Also, the more comfortable we are with our topic, the more effective our speech will be and the less intimidated we will be in front of an audience. Our attitude toward the people in the audience can be influenced by how we feel about them and what we think their reaction to us will be.

DELIVERY

Delivery includes the speaker's style and ability to involve the audience in meaningful learning. The characteristics of an effective public speaker include friendliness, sincerity, the ability to project confidence and be thorough and concise, an awareness of nonverbal messages through body language, and a flexible voice. The nurse should also take into consideration appropriate use of verbal and nonverbal communication, questioning and reinforcement, group interaction, and the use of humor.

Speeches may be memorized or written. Rehearsing, which involves developing an outline, writing notes, and practicing the delivery, increases the effectiveness of the speech. Standing in front of a mirror, audiotaping, and videotaping are also helpful. Remember that over 90% of the message is delivered through voice and body language. Even though audiotaping does not capture body language, it helps to determine whether the speech is too fast or whether the voice is too high in pitch or has a nasal sound. Videotaping can help to identify mannerisms and the use of body language that do not support getting the message across. The wonderful thing about videotaping is that it does not lie; it shows exactly how speakers present themselves. Rehearsing in the room where the speech is to be delivered will improve the speaker's comfort level.

Humor

Humor promotes a relationship between the speaker and the audience. It interests and involves the audience, as well as relaxes them, and people learn better when they are relaxed.

The nurse can integrate humor into a speech in many ways. Using topic-related cartoons, stories, and anecdotes can help emphasize the major points of a presentation. A nurse who is an active public speaker might find it useful to keep a file of humorous stories and pictures.

Humor, such as ethnic jokes, that may offend or alienate members of the audience, should be avoided. It is important to practice telling humorous stories before the presentation. Laughing with and not at others is using healthy humor. Laughing at yourself, especially if a story flops, will put the audience at ease. It is an indication that you are comfortable and self-confident.

INVOLVING THE AUDIENCE

Questioning and Reinforcement

Questioning the audience provides them with an opportunity to show their understanding of the topic. Their responses can help the speaker adjust the delivery and let him or her know how effective the presentation is.

The speaker formulates questions to focus on key points or concepts to make sure that the audience understood them. A question should be stated so that the entire group can respond to it. Allow the audience to volunteer answers rather than selecting members to respond.

When a member of the audience asks a questions, the speaker should always repeat the question so that the entire group can hear it. In this way, the speaker gives recognition to the individual and provides an opportunity to clarify questions and responses.

There are many advantages to questioning. It involves the members of the audience by stimulating and motivating them. The participants have an opportunity to display their understanding of the topic, and to apply the knowledge and skills they have learned. Responses to questions provide feedback to the speaker.

Questioning may be threatening to some members of the audience. They will let the speaker know this by not interacting. Questions can also be time-consuming. Some members of the audience may dominate the discussion and may alienate the rest of the audience.

Feedback

Feedback from the audience lets the speaker know how well the message has been transmitted. One person may be shaking his head in agreement while another has his eyebrow raised. When we speak, we want the audience to receive our message. Audience feedback is usually nonverbal through facial response, eye contact, or laughter in response to humor. When the audience shows interest in the speaker, it strengthens the presentation because the speaker feels more effective and self-confident.

A bored, uninterested audience is responding to an unprepared or unmotivated speaker. This is known as negative feedback. When the speaker presents worthwhile material and shows enthusiasm, the audience will respond with positive feedback.

FORMAL PRESENTATIONS

Preplanning a Presentation

Before a presentation, the nurse should ask the following questions:

1. What are the goals of the presentation?

2. How well do you know the subject area?

3. How will you do the research and preparation?

4. How many people will be attending?

5. How much time will there be for the presentation?

6. Who is the audience? Do they share the same experience and background?

7. Does the audience have any skills or knowledge related to the topic of your presentation?

8. Are participants attending because they are required to attend or is it voluntary?

9. How do the participants learn best— through lecture, demonstration, simulation, group activity, or a combination?

10. Have you developed objectives so the audience can know what they are expected to learn?

11. Will there be a question-and-answer period?

12. Do the participants have special learning needs due to visual, hearing, or mobility deficits?

13. Will you need any audiovisual equipment, such as a slide projector, overhead projector, videoplayer, blackboard, or flip chart?

The answers to these questions will help you structure and plan your presentation, and tailor it to your audience.

Preparing the Setting

Preparing the physical environment is an important part of preparing to speak. For example, even the best speech can fail if the room is overcrowded and hot.

The speaker should arrive well before the audience and check for the following:

1. Locate the temperature and ventilation controls and regulate them so that the climate is appropriate for the audience.

2. Make sure the lighting is adequate. Know where the controls are so that lighting can be adjusted if necessary.

3. Check to see whether the table size is appropriate for the type of activity you have prepared.

4. Test all pieces of audiovisual and demonstration equipment to ensure they are in working order.

5. Check the microphones to make sure they are operating correctly and to adjust the volume.

6. If you are using a blackboard, be sure you have chalk and an eraser.

7. Hang up any posters, charts, or visuals, and make sure they can be seen from anywhere in the room.

8. Bring extra supplies such as writing paper, pens, masking tape, and any other materials you might need.

Effective Behaviors

Certain behaviors can help ensure the success of a presentation. Be sure to do the following:

1. Pay attention to the sound of your voice.

2. Capture the audience's attention by using a strong introduction.

3. Communicate on a personal level.

4. Pronounce and spell words that the audience might find difficult or technical.

5. Write new words on a blackboard or flip chart.

6. Accept and praise ideas shared by audience.

7. Avoid the use of repetitive words such as "okay," "like," "you know." Try not to use "um" or "uh" when pausing.

8. Talk *to*, not *at* your participants. Deliver key words and concepts slowly.

9. Emphasize key points through relevant examples.

10. Use effective body language and facial expressions.

11. Pay attention to unconscious body language that can distract the audience, like jiggling keys or change in your pocket.

12. Demonstrate enthusiasm about your subject and communicate it in your own words.

13. Give clear directions for all activities.

14. Never sit behind a desk or stand behind a lectern, as there should never be a barrier between the speaker and the audience.

15. Use visual aids to illustrate your points.

16. Most importantly, be comfortable and be yourself!

HEALTH EDUCATION

Formal health education is an example of public speaking. It has a structured and planned format with a specific topic and schedule. Advantages of group health education is that the content can be standardized and large numbers of people can be educated. Standardized content must be coordinated by the nurse experts who are planning health education so that a unified approach is presented.

Informal health education is unplanned and spontaneous. Throughout the nurse's workday, there are countless opportunities for health education. Whenever the nurse gives the patient information, the nurse is performing informal teaching. Informal health education may use structured communication.

USING SPEAKING SKILLS

Nurses use public speaking skills in many situations. A change-of-shift report is a common example of a presentation. It is considered routine and informal in some settings, while in other places, it may be formal, along with case presentations, nursing grand rounds, and formal multidisciplinary rounds. Nurses are constantly challenged to use public speaking skills when they present information to patients, physicians, colleagues, administrators, and the lay public.

Nurses can use public speaking skills to communicate an issue or topic they feel strongly about and can practice these skills in many different settings. Nurses can share and develop their talents by providing formal education classes in training and staff development departments. They can teach other nurses by speaking to professional organizations or at a nursing seminar or convention. And nurses can share their knowledge and skills with the community by lecturing to churches, schools, and numerous organizations.

Summary

Public speaking is an important nursing role. In order to be an effective public speaker, the nurse must have professional credibility and the ability to deliver the message. Practicing and preparing for a presentation to suit one's audience is very important. The nurse can incorporate humor into a presentation. It is also important to consider the use of questioning, reinforcement, and feedback. Nurses use public speaking skills in providing formal health education and in many other situations.

Chapter 14

Public Image

Sheila M. Boyle

The word *image* has many definitions, but image as the way in which the nurse is "popularly perceived or regarded" is our focus in this chapter.

WHAT AFFECTS THE NURSE'S IMAGE?

The image of nursing and what the profession can do to improve it have been extensively researched over the past few years. This research indicates that nursing's image can be damaged by TV shows, uncomplimentary advertisements, bad publicity, and by the profession itself. The portrayals of nurses and nursing in television shows have often been unflattering. In fact, the nursing community's outcry resulted in the cancellation of one particular program, in which the nurses spent little time on science courses, wore uniforms that were inappropriate and embarrassing, and were never portrayed caring for patients. The image of the nurse, as perceived by the viewing public, did little to enhance nursing as a career choice. In another TV sitcom, a male nurse received his RN pin by simply following around an office nurse for one day!

When the public is subjected to advertisements in which the nurse is dressed inappropriately, they form a mental image of what a nurse looks like. An ad on our local radio station for an area hospital talks about technology, the skill of the physicians, and "nurses who are there to hold your hand." Is this the message we want to convey to the listening public? Newspapers call anyone who works with patients a "nurse." For example, a nursing technician killed several patients in as many hospitals. The printed stories stated: "nurse kills patients." Imagine the fear such an article generates in those who are anticipating an admission to the hospital in the near future.

The nursing profession itself inspires both positive and negative images. As nurses, we must accept the responsibility of maintaining an image that best states who we are, what we do, and how we are educated. I speak to many high school career classes, and I am always a little bit embarrassed to talk about nursing's educational standards. Imagine explaining to these inquisitive students that a nursing degree can be obtained via three different educational pathways, and that any of the three enables the graduate to take the state board exam that is required to become licensed. The perception by the public might be that the nursing profession cannot seem to agree on how to best educate future nurses. How many other professional careers have so many educational options? As a first step toward improving its image, the nursing community must agree on common educational goals and requirements for the benefit of all present and future nurses.

Why is education such a top priority? If we want smart, capable students to consider a nursing career, we must present a definitive way for them to achieve their goal. Nursing does not offer the financial rewards of other high-profile careers, nor does the 24-hour, 7 days per week operation of hospitals make it a particularly attractive career choice for potential applicants. However, by promising the availability of jobs no matter what hours a nurse can work and the availability of a hospital no matter what community a nurse may live in, the nursing profession can change a perceived negative image to a positive one.

A WOMAN'S WORLD?

The nursing profession is still made up mostly of women. Although women are no longer considered "the weaker sex," there are some who think that female nurses are simply doing a job but male nurses are pursuing a career. This perception exists primarily in the hospital setting where the female nurse is more often observed at the bedside and the male nurse is a manager or nurse anesthetist. I interview male applicants for nursing scholarships and one of the questions asked is "where do you see yourself in five years?" In my six years as a member of this committee, 85 to 90% of the men answer that the RN degree is a stepping stone to specialization or more advanced practice. The female nurse does not seem as goal oriented.

However, the male nurse has his own set of problems in establishing his professional image. The old stereotype that a male is feminine because he has a caring, considerate attitude or that he became a nurse because medical school rejected him is finally changing. Yet when I bring a male applicant to the nursing unit to be interviewed, I still hear remarks like, "Oh good—we need a man to do the heavy lifting." The female nurse needs to examine her attitude and not look at a male colleague as an orderly, but as a valued member of the unit nursing team.

Recently, a male administrator told me that there was little competition for managerial positions in our hospital setting because most of the work force were women who had too many home and child care obligations to take on any more responsibilities. Nurses must change this type of perception if they are to empower themselves in the public's eye. This is an exciting time in health care, with many new ways of delivering care being examined. What better change agent than the bedside nurse who has managed the care of her patients holistically, and understands the need for collaboration with all members of the health care team to affect positive outcomes.

WAYS TO BUILD IMAGE

In order to stay on the leading edge of a very exciting and constantly evolving profession, each nurse must make a decision regarding his or her practice. How nursing is perceived by the public is the responsibility of every nurse in the profession. We must carefully enhance our self-esteem, examine our attitudes, improve our presentation, sharpen our communication skills, serve as mentors to new nurses, become active in our nursing associations and in local community projects (always identify yourself as a nurse!), and make learning a life-long commitment.

Self-Esteem

Nurses should examine how they feel about themselves and their jobs, and remind themselves of their importance. If nurses feel good about who they are and what they do, they appear and will become self-assured, which can have a powerful impact on all facets of their personal and professional lives. Improved self-esteem reflects a positive self-concept, which in turn will enhance our image.

Presentation

To project the image of a professional, nurses need to dress like professionals. Look around your unit and notice how the nurses are dressed—our outfits sometimes look like they were just thrown together. Think about some of the highly respected professionals you come in contact with, such as your physician or lawyer. Are they dressed appropriately when you meet with them? Many patients bemoan the loss of the traditional uniforms and caps that in their eyes signified "nurse." My aunt would not return to an esteemed female neurologist because she examined my aunt in her street clothes. "She didn't even have a lab coat over her dress!"

While it's not our clothes that make us competent and caring, we do need to make sure that what we wear does not send the wrong message. Stand in front of a long mirror before leaving for work and think about what kind of an image you are portraying. Is your uniform of choice opaque (check the panty line), is your jewelry appropriate for performing your job, and are your nails clean, trimmed, and lightly polished? Scrubs are fine if they are clean, ironed, and fit well (not too tight and not too loose). Shoes should be white, polished or unstained, and hose should always be worn. Male nurses have the additional burden of being mistaken as the physician or the orderly, rather than the patient's nurse for the day. They should ensure that their pants, whether uniform or scrubs, are ironed and their nails are clean and trimmed.

Nurses arriving for a personal interview should also be dressed appropriately. I have had to interview men and women in jeans, shorts, and tee shirts with all kinds of writing on them, and one young lady wore a skimpy summer dress cut so low that I didn't know where to look. Presenting yourself in a professional manner lets the interviewer know that you expect to be taken seriously. Proper dress shows that you prepared for the interview, and gives you a distinct advantage over the sloppily dressed candidate.

Communication

Communication is an important component of image. How we speak to patients, co-workers, physicians, and other health care employees reflects how we feel about ourselves and our jobs. Listen attentively at report time and see how we talk about what we do. Do we blame the other shift for things over which they have no control? When we give and get report to and from each other, do we show respect for all that was done, or wait for the change to ask, "Why wasn't this completed?" During my nursing career, I remember fondly those colleagues who would agree to "pick up the ins and outs" or "check the credits on the IVs" when they arrived on the unit to start their shift and saw how busy we were. I also clearly remember the nurses who would go into the nurses lounge and sit waiting for us to finish up—which in reality put them behind! Think back to your last shift report and recall into which category you fit. An extra pair of hands gets everyone back on target, and patient care continues without undue interruption. Blame does not belong on the nursing unit; patient care is a 24-hour commitment, not three separate 8-hour shifts. Don't be guilty of passing on tales about the 3 to 11 or 7 to 3 or 11 to 7 shift. Behaving in a professional manner with each other means that those outside the profession will respect us.

When giving shift report, be cognizant of how you refer to patients: "Did the gall bladder in 178 have pain?" or "Did Mrs. Kresge require post op medication?" When talking to your patients, address them with respect. My 86-year-old grandmother was offended when her nurse called her Katherine. She repeatedly told us that no one called her by her first name except for close friends, and she could not understand how the nurse could be so impertinent and address her in such familiar terms. Ask your patients how they would like to be addressed, and inform other caregivers of these preferences.

Written communication introduces you to your reader. As a nurse recruiter, my first impression of you is through the written word. A sloppily prepared resume will probably mean a lost interview, for it tells me that you did not take the time to research how to prepare a proper resume and therefore you might not be the nurse we are looking for. Articles abound on how to write a resume and an accompanying cover letter. A nurse with a long and impressive list of work experiences sent a cover letter on which misspelled words were "whited out" on buff paper! She applied for the job of Clinical Manager of a busy medical-surgery unit. The position required excellent organizational skills, among other things. She was not considered for the position because of her poorly typed letter.

Role Models

Think back to your first job, and try to remember who your role model was. As a young nurse of twenty, I slept until 10:00 A.M., went out to lunch, and then came back to the nurses home and leisurely prepared for work. I was amazed and impressed by an RN with four children who worked in her home for eight hours before she reported for work at 3:00 P.M. Yet this nurse was always neatly dressed, energetic, willing to answer all my questions, and very caring to her patients. She wore the hats of wife, mother, and nurse equally well, and no one seemed shortchanged. Forty years later, I still refer to her as my first nurse role model. She exhibited the qualities I wanted to emulate as I learned to juggle my personal life and professional career.

Take a look at the new nurses assigned to your unit. Forty years from now, will they remember you as the nurse who was their role model? For this is how a professional image evolves: nurses pass on the positive aspects of a nursing career to all those who follow.

Be a mentor to the new nurses who are struggling to match theory with practice. Be patient with their endless questions, and allay their fears. Take a moment to look back on your career, and see how many trials and errors it took to get where you are now. Be cautious when you are angry and frustrated, so that you don't display negative emotions to those around you. We must care for our colleagues as well as our patients and ourselves.

Community Involvement

Nursing must consider itself to be a community. There is power in numbers, and we should therefore become active members of our local and national organizations. Working with other nurses on issues that affect us will not only strengthen our nursing practice, but will give participants a sense of pride and fulfillment and let others know that we are committed to our profession.

It is also important for nurses who are visible in public. If you volunteer for outside organizations, at school functions, or for any other group, be sure to announce proudly (and loudly) "I am a nurse." My mother always consulted a nurse in our neighborhood before she would take us to the doctor. "Let Mrs. Goode have a look at that rash (cut, etc.)!" I was in awe of this woman who had much knowledge. At that point in my life, my image of nursing was of an intelligent person who seemed to know more than the doctor—even more than my mother.

Education

Continuing education should be a part of every nurse's professional development. I have difficulty understanding nurses who say, "Why should I continue my education? I want to stay at the bedside," or "I don't plan to become a manager." We are members of an ever-changing practice where data on new equipment, new procedures, and treatment modalities are published almost weekly. It is our duty to stay current and up-to-date. If for some reason your formal education must be postponed, study on your own and become certified in your area of practice. Read a current nursing journal, and start a practice on your unit where each month a nurse is responsible for reviewing and reporting on one new article. Be cognizant of current nursing research and how it may affect what we do in the future. Attend as many continuing education offerings as possible, and share what you learned there with others.

Set goals for continuing your education at the undergraduate and graduate levels. Before I was financially able to return to school for my BSN, I would accompany a nurse on my unit to an occasional graduate level nursing course at a prominent university. She would take me to lectures, the book store, and the many stored library, and even received permission for me to observe her as she did a practicum on a heart transplant unit in a large city hospital. This experience showed me that I had so much more to learn about nursing that I began my five-year plan. (It actually took me eight years to complete my BSN, but it was time well spent.) Nurses with master's degrees are gaining more autonomy each year as nurse practitioners or clinical specialists, and some states are now granting them prescriptive practice.

Don't use the excuse that some nurses give me when I encourage them to go back to school: "I'll be fifty years old when I finish." Well, my response is that you'll be fifty years old regardless! One course a semester is a great way to begin. Try to find a buddy to start with you. You can provide each other with encouragement, transportation, notes for classes missed, and a reason to continue.

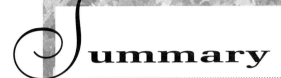

Summary

In this chapter we have discussed what affects the image of nurses. Taking pride in what we do and how we look, being effective in the ways we communicate publicly and with each other, and acquiring more knowledge so our education is ongoing will do much to improve that image. The economy today is demanding change in health care delivery, and nurses must demand to be an integral part of the process. It will take each of us working together and collectively to become part of the solution and not the problem.

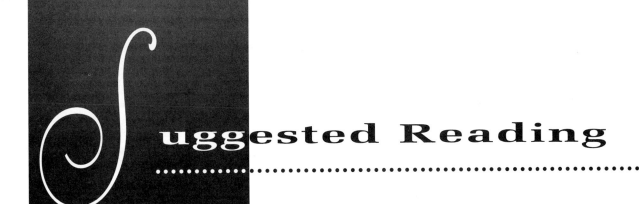

Suggested Reading

Benner, P. *From novice to expert.* Menlo Park, CA: Addison-Wesley, 1984.

Bloch, D. *Words that heal.* New York: Bantam Books, 1990.

Bradley, J. C., & Edinberg, M. A. *Communication in the nursing context.* 3rd ed. San Mateo, CA: Appleton and Lange, 1990.

Buckley, C. D., & Walker, D. *Harmony: professional renewal for nurses.* American Hospital Association Publishing Company, 1989.

Cousins, N. *Anatomy of an illness.* New York: Norton, 1979.

Leebov, W. *Service excellence: the customer relations strategy for health care.* American Hospital Association Publishing Company, 1988.

McKay, M., Davis, M., & Fanning, P. *Messages: the communications skill book.* Oakland, CA: New Harbinger Publications, 1983.

Paulson, T. *Making humor work: take your job seriously and yourself lightly.* Los Altos, CA: Crisp Publications, 1989.

Pattison, R. *The experience of dying.* Englewood Cliffs, NJ: Prentice-Hall, 1977.

Robinson, V. M. *Humor and the health professions.* 2nd ed. Thorofare, NJ: Slack Incorporated, 1991.

Satir, V. *The new peoplemaking.* Mountain View, CA: Science and Behavior Books, 1988.

Sourkes, B. *The deepending shade. Psychological aspects of life-threatening illness.* Pittsburgh: University of Pittsburgh Press, 1982.

Sundeen, S., Stuart, G. W., Rankin, E., & Cohen, S. A. *Nurse-client interaction.* 4th ed. St. Louis: C. V. Mosby, 1989.

Timm, P. R. *Recharge your career and your life.* Los Altos, CA: Crisp Publications, 1990.

Waitley, D. *The joy of working.* New York: Ballantine Books, 1985.

Zahourek, R. P. *Relaxation and imagery: tools for therapeutic communication and intervention.* Philadelphia: W. B. Saunders Company, 1988.

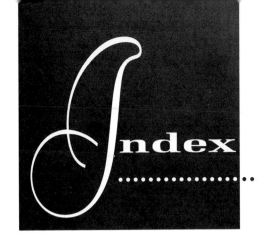

Index

A

Abuse survivors
  handling   86, 89
Accuracy
  interviewing importance   71
  resume importance   150
Action
  generation of, as communication
    goal   9
Advice
  alternatives to giving   76
  communications, problems of   22
  interviewing, error of giving   76
Affirmations
  negative, damaging effects of   31
  positive, effective use of   32
  principles and importance of   30
Agoraphobia
  patient, handling   89
Anger
  active listening role is alleviating   62
  patient, handling   81, 84, 86–87
Anxiety
  active listening role is alleviating   62
  anticipated death, handling   100
  attack, symptoms of   88
  patient, handling   87–90
Apathy
  patient, handling   82
Appearance
  nursing image importance of   150
Arguing
  communications problems of   22
Assertiveness
  reinforcement rewards   4
  visualization role in enhancing   41
Assumptions
  danger of, for interviewing   76

Attitudes

  influencing, as communication goal   8
  relationship of action to   9
Autocratic leader
  characteristics   121

B

Benefits
  effective communication   84
Bereavement
  crisis intervention   97
Blaming
  interviewing error   76
Blocks
  communication   21
Body language
  courteous   81
  empathy component   52
  expressing reassurance with   64–66
  incongruent, as clue to patient
    information discrepancies   74
  nonverbal communication
    characteristics   14–16
Boundaries
  healthy families, characteristics   113
Burnout
  as potential result of
    miscommunication   10
  avoiding, recognition skills for
    avoiding   29

C

Changing the subject
  communications problems of   22
Channel
  communication model component   11

Children
  communicating with   104
Chronic disease
  elderly   106
  families and   112–117
Clarification
  information-gathering
    technique   70, 73
Claustrophobia
  patient, handling   89
Communication
  basic nursing skill   2
  challenges, (chapter)   96–110
  effective   8
  errors, during interviewing   75
  goals   8–10
  humor in, understanding the
    messages   128
  learning methods   3–4
  models, (figure)   10
  nonverbal   14
  nursing image building skill   150–152
  one-way, uses and abuses   11
  outcomes   8–10
  problems, (chapter)   20–26
  situation categories   3
  term definition   2
  theories   16
  two-way   12
  verbal   13
Community involvement
  nursing image building
    component   153
Compassion
  spiritual well-being component   44
Complaints
  patient, handling   81–84
Compliance
  reinforcement rewards   4
Compliments
  importance for effective nursing   29
Confusion
  in the elderly, handling problems
    with   108
Congruence
  communication styles   17
  incongruence, communications
    problems of   23
  lack of, as clue to patient information
  discrepancies   74

nonverbal reassurance importance
  of   65
Controlling
  patient, handling   86
Coping
  with chronic disease, functions
    of   112
Counseling
  importance to patient well-being   25
Courtesy
  as a therapeutic tool   81
Credibility
  role in effective public speaking   140
Crisis
  intervention, characteristics and
    methods   96
Cultural differences
  understanding and handling   117–118

D

Death
  See Dying
Decision-making
  patient, techniques for aiding   76
Decoder
  communication model component   11
Defensiveness
  communications problems of   23
Dehumanization
  interviewing danger when using
    standard forms   70
Demanding
  patient, handling   85
Democratic leader
  characteristics   121
Depression
  in the elderly, handling   106
  patient, handling,   90–93
  primary, handling in patients   92
  reactive, handling in patients   92
  suicide
    intervention procedures   99
    probability assessment   98
Derailing
  communications problems of   22
Discrepancies
  detecting, during interviewing   74
Discrimination
  term definition   4

Displacement
  communication problems   20
Distraction
  communications problems of   24
Dying
  crisis period characteristics   100
  helping children whose parent is   104
  patients, communicating
    with   101–104

E

Education
  importance in building the
    image of nursing   153
Elderly
  communicating with   106
Emotions
  communicating, (chapter)   80–94
  dark, pitfalls in handling   77
  negative, active listening role is
    alleviating   62
  role in miscommunication   9
  self-understanding of, crucial role in
    enhancing ability to listen   64
Empathy
  characteristics and role in effective
    nursing   52
  importance in communicating with
    the dying   101
  importance in handling patient
    complaints   83
  sympathy contrasted with   53
  therapeutic use of, (chapter)   50–58
Encoder
  source, communication model
    component   11
Endorphins
  humor as releaser of   129
Excessive talk
  communications problems of   21
Exploration
  importance for effective
    interviewing   70
Expressive techniques
  mental health role of   39
Extinction
  reinforcement withholding result   4
Eye contact

  interpreting   14
Eyesight
  handling patients with loss of   107

F

Facial expressions
  see also body language
    interpreting   14
False reassurance
  communications problems of   23
Families
  and other groups, (chapter)   112–120
  communicating with   114, 116
  comparison of healthy and
    vulnerable   114
  dying patients, behaviors that
    help   103
  family-systems theory   112
  healthy, characteristics   112
  vulnerable, characteristics   113
Fear
  active listening role is alleviating   62
  in children, handling   105
  in patients, handling   80
  patient, handling   82
Feedback
  communication model component   11
  public speaking, interpreting   142
Filters
  communication problems caused
    by   12
First impressions
  patient communication
    importance   81
Flashbacks
  patient, handling   89
Fluff
  derogatory meaning of   24
Focusing
  information-gathering technique   73

G

Genograms
  usefulness in handling family
    systems   114, 115
Grief
  associated with the anticipation of

dying, handling 100–103
crisis management 97
patient, handling 91
Groups
communicating with 118
dynamics, impact on effectiveness 120
phases of 123–125
power dynamics 123, 124
self-help 122
support, 121, 122
task 119
therapeutic 121

H

Hand gestures
see also body language
interpreting 15
Health education 144
Hearing-impaired
communicating with 106
Helplessness
patient, handling 84–87
High-visibility tasks
characteristics 24
Hope
importance in healing 134
Humanizing
hospital environments, role of
courtesy in 81
Humor
as a positive coping
mechanism 128–133
interventions 130
resources and methods 131, 133
role in effective public speaking 141

I

"I" statements
role in active listening 62
Image, nursing
issues affecting 148
ways to build 150
Imitation
see modeling
Immigrants
classification 117
Incongruence
communications problems of 23
Infants

handling 105
Inferiority
communications, problems of 23
Influence
as communication goal 8
Information gathering
skills, (chapter) 70–78
techniques 71
Intake forms
collecting information with 70
Interaction 12
in public speaking 141
role of active listening in 61
Interpersonal
process, Hidegard Peplau's theory 16
system, Imogene King's theory 17
Interviewing
errors 75
skills, (chapter) 70–78
Irritability
patient, handling 88
Isolation
in the elderly, handling problems
with 107

J

Journal writing
role in enhancing self-esteem 43–45
use in calming mildly anxious
patients, 88
Judging
communications problems of, 21

K

King, Imogene 16
Knowledge
of the patient, importance for
effective nursing 50

L

Laissez-faire leader
characteristics 121
Language
as a communication barrier 117
Leadership styles
groups 121

Leading statements
  as interviewing error   75
Listening
  active, (chapter)   60–68
    effective interviewing   70
    purposes and skills   61
    tips for   67
  empathy component   52
  group leaders   121
  handling patient
    anxiety   88
    complaints   83
  helping dying patients   103
Losses
  grief over, handling in patients   91
Low-visibility tasks
  characteristics   24

M

Macho behavior
  active listening role in decoding   64
Mass communication
  complicating factor in patient care   10
  potential for influence by nurses   9
Meaning
  communication as the process of
    creating   2
Mental health
  self-esteem importance to   39
Messages
  blocks to the communication of   21
  metamessages   20
    problems generated by   20
  whole, versus partial messages   20
Misunderstanding
  emotions role in   9
  resolving, as communication goal   9
Motivation
  importance of understanding   9
Mourning
  patient, handling   91
Movement
  body, interpreting   15
Music
  relaxation role of   43

N

Nonverbal communication   14

  problems generated by   20
  reassurance, appropriate use of   64
Nursing tasks
  communication and   24
  high-visibility tasks   24
  low-visibility tasks   24
  low-visibility tasks vs high-visibility
    tasks   25

O

Objectivity
  importance in handling patient
    complaints   83
Open-ended questions
  information-gathering technique   71
Over-involvement
  dangers and behaviors that indicate
    the presence of   55

P

Panic
  patient, handling   89
Paranoia
  patient, handling   87
Paraphrasing
  information-gathering technique   72
Passivity
  patient, handling   82
Pat on the back
  effective recognition skill   29
Pavlov   3
Peplau, Hildegard   16
Personal
  contact, as a therapeutic tool   81
  system, Imogene King's theory   17
Personality
  patient, characteristic changes   80
Persuasion
  as communication goal   8
Placating
  communications problems of   22
Play therapy
  communicating with children
    through   104
Pleasure
  enhancement of, as communication
    goal   8
Prayer

healing role of 135
Prejudice
  communications problems of 21
Presentations
  delivery guidelines 144
  planning 142
  preparing the setting 143
Preverbal children
  handling 105
Primary failure in communication
  term definition 9
Privacy
  patient, asking questions that seem to
  invade 75
Probing
  information-gathering technique 72
Projection
  patient, handling 86
Psychiatric evaluation
  crisis management use of 97
  primary depression, importance of
  obtaining 92
PTSD (post-traumatic stress disorder)
  patient, handling 89
Public speaking, (chapter) 140–146
  checklist for preparing for 142
  delivery guidelines 144
  effective, components of 140

Q

Questions
  closed-ended, as interviewing error 77
  focused, information-gathering
  technique 73
  open-ended, information-gathering
  technique 71
  role in effective public speaking 141
  sensitive, methods for asking 75
  too many, as interviewing error 77

R

Reassurance
  appropriate use of 64
  as communication goal 8
  false, as interviewing error 77
  negative aspects of 62
Receiver
  communication model component 11

Reflection
  role in active listening 62
Relationships
  balanced 56–57
  improvement, as communication
  goal 9
  over-involvement dangers 55–57
  restructuring to remedy over-
  involvement 57
Relaxation techniques 42
  use in calming mildly anxious
  patients 88
Respect
  See also Image,
  importance in working with the
  elderly 106
  therapeutic tool 81
Role models 152

S

Satir, Virginia 17
Secondary failure in communication
  term definition 9
Self
  images 50
  therapeutic use of 51
Self-defeat
  damaging effects of 31
Self-disclosure
  appropriate versus inappropriate 33
  role in development of trust 54
Self-esteem
  building the image of nursing 150
  effective communications 17
  effective nursing 28–36
  elderly people, importance of
  maintaining 106
  empathy component 52
  evaluation (exercise) 40
  identifying core issues around 42
  lack of feeling of, communications
  problems with 23
  patient, active listening role in
  enhancing 62
  survival 38
Self-help groups
  characteristics 122
Self-knowledge
  critical role in accurate

self-esteem 39
Self-talk
  importance to effective nursing 28
  negative, damaging effects of 28
  positive, importance of 29
Self-worth
  see self-esteem
Selling points
  nursing career 149
Sender
  communication model component 11
Senior citizens
  communicating with 106
Skinner, B.F. 4
Social
  characteristics
    healthy families 112
    vulnerable families 113
  influence, as communication goal 8
  system, relation to nursing, Imogene
    King's theory 17
Socialization
  humor as a tool for 128
Source
  communication model component 11
Spirituality
  enhancing 44–47
  healing role of 134
Standard forms
  collecting information with 70
Standing ovation
  effective recognition skill 29
Stress
  humor as a coping mechanism for
    handling 128
  in patients, handling 80
  role of spiritual well-being in
    reducing 45
  techniques for reducing 38
Style
  role in modeling 5
Suicide
  evaluation of patients for risk of 93
  intervention 98–100
Summarizing
  information-gathering technique 74
Support groups
  characteristics 121
  compared with self-help groups 122
Survival skills

self-care as an important
  component of 38
Sympathy
  empathy contrasted with 53
Systems theory
  families 112

T

Terminally ill
  communicating with 100–103
Terror
  patient, handling 89
Theories
  communication 16
Therapeutic
  groups 121
  role, characteristics of effective 51
Timing
  importance for the success of
    humor 132
  importance in effective
    communications 51
Toddlers
  handling 105
Touch
  expressing reassurance with 66
  loss of sense of, handling patients
    with 107
Trust
  characteristics and development
    of 54
  impediments to the development
    of 55
  therapeutic use of, (chapter) 50–58

U

Understanding
  promotion of, as communication
    goal 8

V

Validation
  use in effective interviewing 70
Verbal communication 13
  difficulties with immigrant
    patients 117

of emotions, active listening role in
  aiding the patient's   63
reassurance, appropriate use of   64
Visual loss
  handling patients with   107
Visualization
  characteristics and role in enhancing
    self-esteem   40
  enhancing spirituality with   134
  techniques   41
Vocal cues
  interpreting   15

W

Well-being
  sense of, insurance, as
    communication goal   8
Writing
  visualization technique   42